THE GODDESS POSE

"Goldberg's book is lots of fun. . . . Even if you don't care enough about yoga to hold a pigeon pose for the length of time it takes to say [the] title, Indra Devi . . . remains no less a fascinating character." —*Los Angeles Times*

"Engaging . . . offers fresh insights into commonly held assumptions, including the relatively new origins of many physical asanas. . . . Goldberg's own discovery of yoga and Indra Devi forms a riveting prologue to an expansive book that underlines how truly global yoga has become [since] it was taken from Indian shores more than a century ago."
—*The Times of India*

"A celebration of female freedom and everything it can bring: an appetite for adventure, fearlessness in the face of challenge, and, most important, discovery and assertion of self."
—Anna Holmes, founding editor, *Jezebel*

"The story of how Devi came to embrace yoga and spread its gospel in America is as fascinating as it is unlikely. . . . [Goldberg's] goal in writing *The Goddess Pose* seems to have been not just chronicling the life of one of the world's great iconoclasts, but also providing a history for how hatha yoga went from an Indian spiritual tradition to an everyday part of western lives. She succeeds admirably on both counts."   —*The Guardian*

"Michelle Goldberg's masterful engagement with her astonishing subject—and with the diverse political, spiritual, and physical worlds she inhabited—is evident on every page."
—Rebecca Traister, author of *Big Girls Don't Cry*

"Goldberg's account of Devi takes the reader through three chronicled, influential centuries of the yogi, actress, and fearless voyager's life which will leave you with a better understanding of how westernized Yoga differs from its roots . . . and a major dose of inspiration to get you on the way to your next blissed-out savasana."   —*Nylon*

"[*The Goddess Pose*] captures Devi's Forrest Gump–like propensity to live parallel to some of the most important moments of the previous century."   —*New York Post*

"[Goldberg] expertly assembles the puzzle pieces of Devi's life, pausing to provide context for the growing influence of spiritualism on modern American life."
—*The Globe and Mail* (Toronto)

"Whether you're a student of yoga, a history buff, an armchair adventurer, or just a reader in search of an unputdownable story that happens to be true, you'll love this fascinating biography of one of the twentieth century's boldest, most influential women."   —Katha Pollitt, author of
Learning to Drive: And Other Life Stories

"Goldberg brings Indra Devi, a complicated and incredible woman, to life in Technicolor brilliance. . . . I'll never think of yoga the same way again—and neither will you."
—Susannah Cahalan,
New York Times bestselling author of *Brain on Fire*

"Terrific. . . . An irresistible story of yoga's unlikely and, yes, even audacious origins."   —*BookPage*

Michelle Goldberg

THE GODDESS POSE

Michelle Goldberg is a journalist and the author of the *New York Times* bestseller *Kingdom Coming: The Rise of Christian Nationalism*, which was a finalist for the New York Public Library's Helen Bernstein Book Award for Excellence in Journalism, and *The Means of Reproduction: Sex, Power, and the Future of the World*, winner of the J. Anthony Lukas Work-in-Progress Award and the Ernesta Drinker Ballard Book Prize. A senior contributing writer at *The Nation*, she has also written pieces for *The New Yorker*, *The New York Times*, *Newsweek*, *The New Republic*, *Glamour*, and many other publications. She lives in Brooklyn with her husband and children.

www.michellegoldberg.net

THE
GODDESS
POSE

THE GODDESS POSE

The Audacious Life of

INDRA DEVI

the Woman Who Helped Bring Yoga to the West

MICHELLE GOLDBERG

VINTAGE BOOKS

A Division of Penguin Random House LLC | New York

FIRST VINTAGE BOOKS EDITION, MAY 2016

Copyright © 2015 by Michelle Goldberg

All rights reserved. Published in the United States by Vintage Books, a division of
Penguin Random House LLC, New York, and distributed in Canada by Random House
of Canada, a division of Penguin Random House Canada Limited, Toronto. Originally
published in hardcover in the United States by Alfred A. Knopf, a division of
Penguin Random House LLC, New York, in 2015.

Vintage and colophon are registered trademarks of Penguin Random House LLC.

The Library of Congress has cataloged the Knopf edition as follows:
Goldberg, Michelle.
The goddess pose : the audacious life of Indra Devi, the woman who helped bring yoga
to the West / Michelle Goldberg.
pages cm
Includes bibliographical references and index.
1. Devi, Indra, 1899–2002.   2. Yogis—United States—Biography.
3. Hatha yoga.   I. Title.
B132.Y6D4754 2015   613.7'046092—dc23   [B]   2014033125

Vintage Books Trade Paperback ISBN: 978-0-307-47744-6
eBook ISBN: 978-1-101-87464-6

Book design by Maggie Hinders

www.vintagebooks.com

Printed in the United States of America
10   9   8   7   6

To Zev and Lucie

Query: how to combine belief that the world is to a great extent illusory with belief that it is none the less essential to improve the illusion? How to be simultaneously dispassionate and not indifferent, serene like an old man and active like a young one?

—*Eyeless in Gaza*, ALDOUS HUXLEY

CONTENTS

THE
GODDESS
POSE

NEVER WOULD have started doing yoga if there had been aerobics in the Himalayas, but I was desperate.

The few times I'd taken yoga classes in college, my failed attempts to relax redoubled my anxiety. Each pose was a reminder of the lifelong inflexibility that had often mortified me. When I was a little girl, a sadistic ballet teacher barred me from a holiday party because of my terrible splits. In elementary school, I dreaded being forced to sit "Indian style," because it left my hips and back screaming. Later, trying yoga, my awkward efforts to keep my legs and back straight while touching my toes and my inability to do even a half lotus only left me tense and humiliated, convinced that the practice was best for those who were already calm, willowy, and graceful.

Besides, while I'd been captivated by India's kaleidoscopic religious richness during months of traveling, I was wary of anyone purporting to peddle enlightenment to credulous Westerners. On my first trip to the country, a short backpacking sojourn in the late 1990s, I'd read and loved Gita Mehta's *Karma Cola*, a wry Indian look at the Western spiritual tourists who flock to the subcontinent, and the enterprising Indian sages who've risen to meet the demand. "As our home industry expands on every front, at last it is our turn to mass market," she writes. The hippie spiritual scene interested me as a journalistic subject, but I certainly didn't want to participate in it. I wasn't sure if I could even chant "Om" with a straight face.

Yet, I needed exercise. Living in McLeod Ganj, a mountain village just outside the city of Dharamsala, where the Tibetan exile movement was headquartered, I was sick of hiking. My husband and I—we'd eloped the previous year, when I was twenty-four and he was twenty-eight—were about six months into what would be a year-long trip through Asia. Prior to our departure, he'd worked at an Internet start-up. When he cashed out his stock options before they bottomed out in the crash of the late 1990s, we became Internet thousandaires, with a sum in the low five figures that seemed, at the time, to be a fortune. Both of us loved to travel. Putting all our stuff in storage, we flew to Ho Chi Minh City.

After three months bumming around Southeast Asia, we went from Singapore to the tip of the Indian state of Tamil Nadu, then west to the relatively idyllic state of Kerala, where, while lying on a beach, we were approached by movie producers looking for extras for an Indian musical. They were shooting a scene in an ashram, and since no Indian ashram is complete without a handful of flaky Westerners, they asked for our help. Delighted, we agreed. On set, we met a thirty-two-year-old Argentine devotee of the real-life guru Sai Baba, about whom I'd long been curious. His followers believe he's God, and I'd seen his face, beaming beneath his surprising Afro, on stickers and trinkets for sale all over the country. A former medical student, the Argentine had given up her studies and her Buenos Aires apartment after dreaming that Sai Baba summoned her to India.

Later, as we snaked our way north, we visited her at Sai Baba's enormous Prasanthi Nilayam ashram, in a barren corner of Andhra Pradesh, one of India's poorest states. The ashram boasted a shiny planetarium, two hospitals that treated patients for free, a college, a music school, and a brand-new airport for wealthier devotees with private planes. Around the edges, luxury apartment buildings were replacing mud huts. Rather than requesting two of the ashram's ten thousand beds, we checked into a nearby hotel. Every afternoon, a loudspeaker piped in music praising the guru. When I bought a pen at a local shop to take notes, it had Sai Baba's smiling face on it.

There was an ambient spiritual hysteria at Prasanthi Nilayam. At dinner one evening, a devotee we'd become friendly with pointed out an Austrian woman tugging her listless seven-year-old son behind her. She was in the midst of a spiritual crisis because she'd had a dream in which Sai Baba instructed her to abandon the boy and live on the streets as a beggar, and she didn't know if she had the "strength" to do it. As far as I could tell, no one at the ashram was stepping forward to discourage her.

I also heard rumors of sexual abuse and was shocked to meet old hands at the ashram who accepted these stories as true, though they interpreted the molestations as part of Sai Baba's divine mission. One man, an American ex-motivational speaker, thought they were part of Baba's plan to spread his message. "Probably more people are going to know about you if there are allegations that you're a pedophile than if you say God is incarnated on earth," he told me. I ended up writing a story about all this for *Salon*. It didn't leave me any more eager to find a guru.

Arriving in McLeod Ganj, weeks later, my husband and I saw a flyer seeking volunteers to teach English at a school for Tibetan refugees. After months of lassitude, we were thrilled and relieved at the chance to be useful and threw ourselves into the work. Settling down for several months in the sweet, peaceful little town, blessedly cool after months on the roasting plains, I realized I needed to get in shape. Most travelers who wander around India on the cheap lose weight, but I have an iron stomach, as well as a weakness for nan and paneer tikka masala. There was a three-hour ashtanga-based yoga class that met early every morning in a gymnasium near the center of town, and I signed up for it.

It was excruciating. I didn't know it at the time, but ashtanga was initially based on exercise routines developed for teenage boys. The jump-backs we did between poses—like squat-thrusts followed by half push-ups—were channels for an animal energy I'd never possessed. The contortions required for binding poses were out of reach, the inversions terrifying, and I still couldn't do a split, but I kept going back, at first because I wanted to lose weight, then because my friends in town were also going, and finally because it left me feeling fantastic.

A lot of the credit goes to my teacher, Vijay, a Gumby-limbed South Indian who could toss his ankle behind his neck as casually as if he were flinging a scarf. Vijay had very few pretensions. Once, catching me smoking a cigarette, he plucked it out of my fingers—and then started puffing on it himself. "Vijay, what are you doing? You're a yogi!" I cried. "Michelle," he said to me with a gleam in his eye, "I'm not a yogi. I'm a businessman." I appreciated this sort of candor.

Before I left India, Vijay said to me, "Smoking won't interfere with your yoga, but yoga will interfere with your smoking." This turned out to be true; a year later, I quit. By then, my husband and I were living in Brooklyn. I was working as a journalist and writing about politics, which often left me knotted and angry. Yoga became a refuge. Sometimes I practiced four or five times a week. In the ritual and community of classes, I began to sense some of the consolation that others find in religion. Though still not a believer in anything supernatural, I felt the benefits of stepping outside the rush of ordinary life and trying to attune myself to a higher state of consciousness, however inchoate and fleeting. The discipline of paying attention to the habitual way your thoughts unfold, to the familiar grooves of your mind, seemed like cognitive therapy, but cheaper. I loved that I could find psychological solace and a workout at the same time.

I would never be lithe or supple, but I learned to do things with my body that I hadn't thought possible. Occasionally, I would even feel that there was something positive in the tedious loathing I'd always felt for my never-skinny frame, since without that loathing, I might never have taken up yoga in the first place.

But while I loved yoga, I also wondered about it. The claims made for the curative powers of certain poses—the idea that one specific arrangement of limbs could treat depression, another fight headaches or PMS—seemed almost magical. I cringed at the way some of my American teachers romanticized India, a country that, for all its religious magnificence, can also be a place of staggering brutality. And I knew that despite descriptions of postural yoga as a quintessentially Indian discipline, the sweaty, fast-paced style I was practicing in New York was hard to find outside of tourist enclaves on the subcontinent. Everyone in my yoga class back in McLeod Ganj had been from the United States, Europe, Australia, or Israel. Vijay told me his own teacher had been a Frenchman. The Indian yogis I encountered, by contrast, tended to be dreadlocked mendicants practicing torturous physical austerities—standing on one leg for days, sleeping on a bed of nails—that seemed a universe away from anything one learns in a modern yoga class.

Among Western yogis, the standard explanation for the relative scarcity of their style of yoga in India is that most Indians have lost touch with their heritage. Still, I was curious what exactly the connection was between the ash-covered sadhus I'd seen contorting themselves on the banks of the Ganges in Benares and the invigorating stretches, lunges, twists, and handstands I practiced first in McLeod Ganj and then in ninety-minute sessions on a rubber mat in Brooklyn. I started looking around for a book or an article that would explain it. And at some point, I came across the *New York Times* obituary for Indra Devi.

"Indra Devi, the daughter of European nobility who introduced the ancient discipline of yoga to the Kremlin leadership, Hollywood stars like Gloria Swanson and even students in India, died on Thursday in Buenos Aires," the obit began. "She was 102." The piece explained that she'd learned from the same guru as B. K. S. Iyengar and K. Pattabhi Jois, yoga masters I'd heard about from serious students in India. It described her life as a Berlin cabaret performer and an actress in early Indian cinema. According to the obituary, she taught "what was thought to be the first yoga class in modern China" and wrote the first book on yoga by a Westerner to be published in India.

In Indra Devi's story, I thought, I'd find the answers I was looking for. So I began to trace the path of her strange, occasionally inscrutable, and often epic life. As I'd hoped, that life does indeed give us a way to understand where yoga as we practice it in the West came from, showing both its links to an ancient Indian tradition and its wild discontinuities. It reveals how the discipline has been shaped by long dialogue among India, Europe, and America. In a strange way, following the serpentine tale of Devi's life and teachings resolved whatever anxiety I had had about modern yoga's authenticity, because it showed that there's never been a pristine, eternal tradition to corrupt.

The narrative of Devi's life, however, is much more than the story of yoga in the West. As I dove into it, I felt that I was discovering a secret sideways history of the twentieth century. Devi was a Zelig-like figure, an esoteric female Forrest Gump who seemed to show up wherever tumultuous world events were unfolding. Her story moves through the Russian Revolution, the cabarets of Weimar Berlin, the Indian independence movement, the World War II Japanese occupation of Shanghai, and Hollywood during its 1950s heyday. She pops up, somewhat randomly, in Dallas when JFK was shot and then in Saigon when the Vietnam War was raging. That ashram I visited in Andhra Pradesh? It turns out that she was the one who spread Sai Baba's fame across the West. She crossed paths with Gandhi, Greta Garbo, and John Lennon. As spiritual adviser to Manuel Noriega's second-in-command, her name appears in most histories of the U.S. invasion of Panama.

It's an astonishing story, and once I started trying to write it, I realized why no one had told it before. What source material exists is scattered in archives, old newspapers, government files, and friends' houses all over the world. Some is in English, but some is in Russian, Czech, German, Polish, and Spanish, and the last is the only one of the languages in which I have any facility. Devi published several books, including, when she was one hundred, a Spanish-language memoir titled *Una mujer de tres siglos*, or "A Woman of Three Centuries." Her autobiographical writing, however, is highly selective, full of large gaps. In her memoir, there are fewer than eight pages about her eight years in China. Some important incidents are ignored entirely.

In parts of this book, I had no choice but to use Devi's own version of events as my guide. But I also dug up old letters and mentions of her in out-of-print books. I obtained her confidential FBI file—J. Edgar Hoover, not surprisingly, had his eye on her—and the service record of her diplomat first husband. I hired a researcher to help me navigate archives in Riga, Latvia, where she was born, and in Berlin. In addition to those countries, I traveled to India, Argentina, Mexico, and Panama. I spent a lot of money on professional translators, sometimes not knowing whether the material would be useful until after I read it in English. Even after all this, lacunae remain. Most of the people who knew Devi in life found her, on some level, ungraspable, and she remains elusive in death.

This is partly because she had so many identities. Again and again, she would build a life for herself and then discard it when it no longer suited, moving on with no discernable effort or regret. You can see her talent for rebirth in how often she changed her name. Born Eugenia Peterson, she was also known as Eugenie and Jane, and later Indira and Indra, all in combination with various surnames. For her, constant openness to change was a spiritual precept, though it also marks her as a very modern sort of celebrity. (In the pages that follow, I will refer to her as Eugenia until she arrives in Hollywood and officially becomes Indra Devi.)

Many people who knew her spoke to me, including two close friends who themselves had tried, unsuccessfully, to write the story of her life, and who generously shared everything they'd learned. (A writer named Natalia Apostolli was finally able to produce a Spanish-language biography of Devi in 1992. Titled *Una vida, un siglo*, or "One Life, One Century," it is based almost entirely on Devi's stories and recollections.)

Some of those who loved her and who helped me will be disappointed in this book. To them, she was nearly divine. I see her as a complicated, audaciously modern, sometimes inspiring, and sometimes maddeningly irresponsible woman, not as a spiritual exemplar.

Indeed, the more I learned about Devi, the more I doubted that her ethic of nonattachment, an idea often bandied about in yoga classes, was truly compatible with passionate loyalty to other people. In "Reflections on Gandhi," published a year after the Mahatma's assassination, George Orwell writes, "In this yogi-ridden age, it is too readily assumed that 'non-attachment' is . . . better than a full acceptance of earthly life . . . If one could follow it to its psychological roots, one would, I believe, find that the main motive for 'non-attachment' is a desire to escape from the pain of living, and above all from love, which, sexual or non-sexual, is hard work." This opinion is reductive, but after spending years researching Devi's life, which is in many ways a triumph of nonattachment, I don't think Orwell was entirely wrong.

Yet yoga remains as important to me as ever. My yoga classes even helped me deal with the doubts about yoga that occasionally emerged while I was writing this book. I think this is why the practice is such a comfort to secular urbanites like me—it's a technique, not a faith. You don't have to believe in anything, even yoga itself, to find joy and solace in the conscious joining of breath and movement, or relief in slowing the whirling of the mind. You just have to do it.

Devi played a huge role in teaching the world to do yoga. For that, I'm not only fascinated by her, but also grateful. She, more than any cave-dwelling ascetic or Brahmin sage, is the godparent of a practice that has had an enormous impact on contemporary culture as well as on my own wholly worldly life.

PART I

EUGENIA

NDRA DEVI had two husbands and several paramours, but the great elusive love of her life was her mother. In stories about Devi's childhood and adolescence, her mother is like a magical fairy, appearing suddenly, radiating glamour and adventure, and then disappearing just as quickly. Later, during the years after the Russian Revolution, Devi seemed to be forever searching for her through the cities of the disintegrating empire, following rumored sightings of her mother from place to place, occasionally catching up with her and her bohemian friends, and then losing her again.

Devi distrusted psychoanalysis and never, even in her last years, dwelled on the past. She would have recoiled at the idea that her mother had wounded her in any serious way. Instead, she insisted that her mother showed her the importance of independence and of pursuing one's passion. "As a child, I intuited that happiness only came to those that dared to follow their own path," Devi writes. "I forged myself as an independent being, and I was never tied to a place, nor a religion." She often spoke about the necessity of balancing love and detachment, a lesson she learned as much from her mother as from her later Indian gurus.

Yet, while it's true that Devi's mother bequeathed her the spirit of freedom, Eugenia's childhood was also marked by stretches of loneliness, loss, and terror, emotions that sent the young girl searching for spiritual comfort. There's an inadvertently heartbreaking moment in her memoir when she recalls being arrested and imprisoned with her mother after sneaking across a frozen river forming the Russian and Polish borders. It's sad not because Eugenia was traumatized by captivity but because she found it, somehow, sweet. Finally, she writes, she and her mother had the opportunity to connect, to talk at length and support each other through their difficulties.

Sasha Zitovich, a sixteen-year-old Russian aristocrat, gave birth to Eugenia Vassilievna in the spring of 1899 in the Latvian city of Riga, then part of the Russian Empire. According to the old-fashioned Julian calendar that was used in Russia before the revolution, Eugenia's birthday was May 12 (April 30 on the Gregorian calendar we use today). Her father was Vasili Pavlovich Peterson, a middle-aged banker of Swedish origin. Evidently Sasha's father, Count Vasili Mijailovich Zitovich, thought that Peterson offered stability for his strong-willed daughter. Yet the marriage quickly fell apart, and not long after Eugenia's first birthday, her mother and father separated, and Sasha returned to her father's house.

At the time, Eugenia was already living with her grandparents. Sasha had allowed them to nurse her daughter through an infant illness, and week after week, they begged Sasha to let the baby stay just a little longer. Eventually, for reasons that aren't entirely clear, it was decided that Eugenia would remain permanently with Sasha's parents, and they coddled her through her infancy.

A member of the czar's administration, Eugenia's grandfather worked for the police department, and the family lived in a stately home attached to one of the department's district headquarters. It was a grand three-story brick building in a bucolic part of the city, by the Daugava River, which at the time was clean enough for swimming. The building is still standing, though today it's abandoned, carpeted inside with garbage, its façade adorned with graffiti, the area around it desolate. Back then, though, cobblestone streets and small wooden houses surrounded it. To Eugenia, it seemed a grand mansion.

Riga was then a cosmopolitan and quickly growing city, the largest in the Baltics, with communities of ethnic Latvians, Russians, Germans, Poles, Lithuanians, and Jews. Its port was one of the most important in the Russian Empire, a hub for the trade of both raw materials and delicacies from European colonies—coffee, cocoa, spices, fruits. All sorts of European languages were heard in the streets. The city was highly literate, with as many as two hundred places to buy books and a vibrant and rapidly expanding theater scene, nurtured by local artists and visiting performers from Moscow, St. Petersburg, and Berlin. Across the river from the Zitovich home, gorgeous Art Nouveau buildings were being erected on the city's broad avenues, their ornate façades decorated with flowers, angels, gargoyles, and goddesses.

For Sasha, trapped at home, her romantic life officially over before she'd turned eighteen, the urban ferment on the other side of the Daugava must have been a constant temptation, and her existence with her family stifling. But Devi remembered life in her grandparents' house as a perpetual celebration. There was a constant stream of guests, endless parties and receptions. Summers were spent in Jūrmala, a nearby spa town fronting a long, sandy beach.

Not long after Sasha's arrival, Sasha's sister, Marusia, fled her own unhappy marriage to join them, bringing her baby son, Nicolas, with her and providing Eugenia with a permanent playmate. Eugenia had no chores; servants did all the housework. Her adoring grandfather lavished her with dolls and dresses. He was strict only about her studies, so much so that by the time she started school at age ten, she could already read German and French in addition to Russian.

Eugenia's father had completely vanished from her life; she didn't even know what he looked like. One time, her nanny showed her a photo of the famed Russian opera singer Leonid Sobinov and said that he was her father. Her grandmother later disabused her of this; still, whenever Eugenia thought of her father, Sobinov's darkly handsome, dreamy-eyed image came to mind. She wasn't particularly bothered by his absence—if anything, she feared the prospect of one day being forced to meet him, a virtual stranger.

Yet when her mother disappeared, that was agonizing. Sasha had always dreamed of becoming an actress, but her father found the idea of his daughter onstage intolerable. In aristocratic circles, acting was considered a thoroughly disreputable profession, barely a step above prostitution. She was determined, though, and one night when Eugenia was a small child, Sasha packed a bag and ran away from home, joining a small touring theater company in another city.

In her memoir, Devi says that even then she admired her mother for "going totally against the conventions of the epoch and doing what her heart dictated." Yet with her mother gone, she was plagued by inexplicable terrors and constant anxiety. She was afraid of death, afraid that her mother would die, terrified that her nanny would abandon her. An organ grinder used to visit her grandfather's house with his pet monkey, who carried a red bag and wore a military hat. In Eugenia's macabre dreams, the monkey became a murderous beast. The silhouette of a basket floating in the Daugava River looked to her like a corpse. Worst of all was the sight of coffins, which paralyzed her with an overwhelming, lifelong fear of being buried alive.

Sasha had little contact with her family until a serious illness brought her own mother, Eugenia's grandmother, to her hospital bedside. There was a rapprochement, and Sasha's parents grudgingly accepted her stage career. After that, Sasha would return home when she wasn't touring, thrilling her daughter. She'd adopted the stage name Alexandra Labunskaia, and Eugenia saw her as a great star. This was probably an exaggeration, though it is doubtless Sasha had admirers. Whereas Eugenia would always be slight, her mother was broad shouldered and fashionably zaftig, with full lips and a direct, flirtatious gaze. A review of one of her performances praised her "décolleté," while another noted her enticing "coquettish gestures."

Like many aristocratic girls, Eugenia was educated at home, though she longed to go to school. In the afternoons, she would sit by the window and listen with envy to the voices of children returning from their studies. Finally, her ceaseless pleading to her grandparents paid off, and when she was ten, she was enrolled in secondary school. There she insisted that she was Eugenia Labunskaia, not Peterson, and that no one was to call her by her father's surname. It was the first of what were to be many reinventions.

She loved school, and most subjects save mathematics came easy to her—though, just to be sure, she and her friends would eat five-petal lilacs before exams, a superstition meant to ensure good grades. After classes, Eugenia would walk home with her best friend, Nina Tretiakovy, and Nina's older brother Vava, who went to school nearby. Eugenia loved their big, lively house, where the kids (seven in all) seemed to have the run of the place. Though generally shy, there she was uninhibited. Vava always had a talent for wordplay, and he would sit at the piano improvising funny songs while Nina and Eugenia danced along.

No one would have guessed that Eugenia, alternately insecure and headstrong, would one day be admired as a spiritual leader. If anything, she was a bit of a brat, furiously impatient when forced to wait for her servants to clean or iron her clothes. For an aristocratic only child, perhaps this wasn't unusual, but looking back almost a century later, she writes, "I also want it known that I recognize myself as terribly human, with all the debilities belonging to humanity. I don't have a trace of sainthood."

In the summer of 1910, Eugenia's nanny took her and her cousin, Nicolas, to visit her mother in Sevastopol, a Crimean resort city on the Black Sea. Eugenia thrilled to witness the fans who came to stand outside her mother's hotel window, the delirious applause at the theaters, and the heaps of proffered flowers onstage.

As Eugenia entered adolescence, the cozy, protective world of her childhood began to fall apart. Her grandfather had a stroke and died when she was twelve, and the constant anxiety that plagued her intensified. Nicolas departed for military school, returning on holidays transformed from a sweet companion into a swaggering, supercilious bully who enjoyed humiliating her by belting out obscene songs. As she lost those around her, her mother's visits became more and more important to her. Eugenia loved to stand by her side at the piano in her family's salon, luxuriating in the timbre of her mother's voice.

In her early teens, Eugenia was allowed to visit Sasha when she was performing in Moscow. They would stay at the famed Hotel Metropol, a sumptuously decorated Art Nouveau palace full of gothic pinnacles and soaring atriums, with ultramodern conveniences such as telephones and hot running water. In the evenings they'd sometimes visit the nearby Bolshoi Theatre. Eugenia remembered the excitement of strolling hand in hand through the city with Sasha, stopping at restaurants and bohemian cafés, and being delighted when strangers recognized her mother. Walking beside Sasha, her own bearing proud and her chin aloft, she felt like a bit of a star herself.

It was in Moscow, during the winter of 1914, that Eugenia first came across the word *yoga*. World War I had started that July, and on the front, Russian soldiers were dying by the hundreds of thousands. Yet such suffering seemed far away. In Moscow, sleighs plied the snowbound streets, and Eugenia would accompany her mother on afternoon visits to the homes of friends, where they'd drink tea for hours before crackling fires.

One day, at the house of one of her mother's actor friends, Eugenia slipped away and found his enormous library, with volumes crammed onto floor-to-ceiling bookshelves. On a desk were two that seemed particularly well thumbed. One was by the Indian poet and novelist Rabindranath Tagore, who had, the previous year, become the first South Asian to win the Noble Prize in Literature. The second was *Fourteen Lessons in Yogi Philosophy and Oriental Occultism*, by Yogi Ramacharaka.

As the title promises, the book deals more with philosophy and occultism than physical practice; one of its chapters is subtitled "Clairvoyance, Clairaudience, Psychometry, Telepathy, etc.—How to Develop Psychic Powers." It does, however, offer a tantalizing hint of the discipline that would reshape Eugenia's life. "The care of the body, under the intelligent control of the mind, is an important branch of yogi philosophy, and is known as 'Hatha Yoga,'" Rama-charaka writes. "We are preparing a little text-book upon 'Hatha Yoga,' which will soon be ready for the press, that will give the Yogi teachings upon this most important branch of self-development."

Just as Eugenia sat down to read Ramacharaka's book, her mother's friend entered the room. "Aha! I see that you have discovered the most precious book in my collection," he said. And taking the book from her, he began to read. The dancing light of a nearby fire flickered in the room, and as the actor pronounced the strange, mysterious words, Eugenia's cheeks burned. Suddenly, surprising herself with her own ardor, she announced, "I have to go to India!"

With a wary look, he closed the book. "You are too emotional, my dear," he said.

Actually, the author of *Fourteen Lessons in Yogi Philosophy and Oriental Occultism* wasn't from India. Yogi Ramacharaka was a nom de plume of William Walker Atkinson, who lived in Chicago. Atkinson was a leading proponent of New Thought, a kind of proto-self-help movement that claimed that the power of the mind could control external events. His books included *Thought Force in Business and Everyday Life* and *Dynamic Thought; or, the Law of Vibrant Energy*. When he published his book about hatha yoga, the exercises he described hardly resembled traditional asanas, or yoga poses. "Swing back the hands until the arms stand out straight . . . The arms should be swung with a rapid movement, and with animation and life. Do not go to sleep over the work, or rather play," he writes.

It was fitting that his book should fall into Eugenia's hands, since the strange coupling of Indian spirituality and Occidental self-improvement was to be a major theme in her life.

Such a book wasn't out of place in the library of a Russian actor of the time. Russia's Silver Age, an extraordinarily rich, romantic period of artistic innovation that began around the turn of the twentieth century, was saturated with spiritualism, Eastern religion, and esoteric magic. "The shelves of the Russian philosophical bookshops of that day abounded in works on Oriental mysticism, Buddhism, Vedanta and Yoga, when Western Europe still had but scant acquaintance with these subjects," writes Sir Paul Dukes, a famed British spy and yoga aficionado whose own metaphysical explorations began in prerevolutionary Riga and St. Petersburg.

Between 1881 and 1918, more than eight hundred occult books appeared in Russia. The work of Papus, a leading French occultist, was widely available, and he became a significant adviser to Czar Nicholas and Czarina Alexandra (though nowhere nearly as important to them as the debauched monk Rasputin). In St. Petersburg, hundreds turned out for Theosophical lectures at the Tenishev School, a prestigious private secondary school—Vladimir Nabokov was enrolled there—with one of the best auditoriums in the city.

Of all the esoteric spiritual associations flourishing in Russia during Eugenia's adolescence, Theosophy, the grandmother of today's New Age movements, was the most widespread, particularly among elites. Though born in America, it had Russian roots: Helena Petrovna Blavatsky, its founder, was, like Eugenia, the child of Russian aristocrats. Madame Blavatsky, as she was called, was a fat, chain-smoking, riotously vulgar spiritualist, usually dressed in shapeless black clothes and bedecked with shawls and baubles. Her father was a Russian soldier descended from a family of minor German nobles; her mother, from a more august line, was a novelist and early feminist. By the time Blavatsky arrived in the United States via Paris in 1873, the story she told about her life was a glittery farrago of the factual and fantastical. It's a fact that in 1849, when she was seventeen, she married Nikifor Blavatsky, vice governor of Yerevan in the Caucasus, and that she fled from him a few months later, choosing to set off alone for Constantinople rather than return to her father. After that, myth and history become more entangled.

Blavatsky claimed to have traveled the world studying with various spiritual teachers, including Sufi *pirs*, Egyptian Kabbalists, voodoo priests in New Orleans, and, most important, a Tibetan by the name of Master Morya, with whom, she said, she'd apprenticed in the Himalayas for seven years. In between, there were more worldly adventures. In his splendid book *Madame Blavatsky's Baboon*, historian Peter Washington writes that she professed "to have ridden bareback in a circus, toured Serbia as a concert pianist, opened an ink factory in Odessa, traded as an importer of ostrich feathers in Paris, and worked as interior decorator to the Empress Eugénie." She had scars that she claimed came from fighting alongside Giuseppe Garibaldi, the Italian revolutionary hero. She supported herself, in part, as an itinerant clairvoyant. "She may or may not have had lovers," writes Washington, "including the German Baron Meyendorf, the Polish Prince Wittgenstein and a Hungarian opera singer, Agardi Metrovich." She may have given birth to one or two illegitimate children, though, if she did, their whereabouts are unknown.

Arriving in New York, Blavatsky sought to establish herself as a medium. By most accounts, her belief in the reality of hidden worlds and esoteric secrets was sincere, but she was also canny, ambitious, and more than willing to engage in tricks to convince others of her abilities. For a woman with few resources save eclectic religious knowledge, charisma, and bravado, spiritualism offered rare and potentially lucrative career opportunities. It was one of the few fields where women, thought to possess greater intuition than men, were at an advantage.

In the United States, Blavatsky soon joined forces with Henry Steele Olcott, an agricultural expert, lawyer, Civil War veteran, and journalist. Olcott was a successful and established man—he was a member of the three-man board appointed to investigate Abraham Lincoln's assassination. It's less surprising than it might seem that he would get involved with Blavatsky. At the time, many serious people took spiritualism seriously. In 1854, Senator James Shields, a Democrat from Illinois, presented a petition on the Senate floor, signed by fifteen thousand American spiritualists, demanding a "scientific commission" to investigate communication with the dead. Spiritualism continued to grow after the American Civil War, fed by people's desperation to hear from their lost loved ones. First Lady Mary Lincoln held séances at the White House in an attempt to contact her dead son. Major newspapers ran dispatches about spiritual manifestations.

One evening in September 1875, a small group, including Olcott, gathered in the parlor of Madame Blavatsky's apartment on Irving Place in Manhattan. They were there to hear a lecture on something called "The Lost Canon of Proportion," a kind of esoteric Egyptian geometry. (In the Western imagination, Egypt preceded India as a seat of mysterious secret wisdom, and Kabbalah-inspired speculation about quasi-magical mathematical formulas was popular in many occultist circles.)

As Olcott later reported it, during the lecture, the idea of a group devoted to investigating ancient mysteries, secret societies, and magic occurred to him spontaneously. He passed Blavatsky a note suggesting it, she agreed, and he proposed it to the whole room. "I dwelt upon the materialistic tendencies of the age and the desire of mankind to get absolute proof of immortality; pointing to the enormous spread of the spiritualistic movement as the best evidence of that fact," he writes. Everyone agreed, and the Theosophical Society was born.

By the end of November, the Theosophical Society had adopted bylaws and elected officers. Olcott was president, while Blavatsky was corresponding secretary (and unofficial sage). The group devoted itself to a threefold purpose: promoting the brotherhood of man, studying comparative religion, and investigating "the unexplained laws of Nature and the powers latent in humanity." These aims were vague enough to encompass all sorts of people, and Theosophy attracted freethinkers and liberal Christian clergy as well as spiritualists.

Blavatsky and Olcott rented an apartment on West Forty-Seventh Street that served as her home and their headquarters and salon. It was a shambolic, extravagantly decorated place that journalists jokingly called "the Lamasery." Besides its plush Victorian furniture, Persian rugs, profusion of Asian icons and ornaments, and tumbling piles of books and papers, the space was notable for the many taxidermist's animals scattered about, most strikingly a bespectacled baboon in a shirt and tie. The baboon carried under its arm a manuscript of a lecture on Darwin; as Peter Washington notes, it stood for "the Folly of Science as opposed to the Wisdom of Religion."

Yet the Theosophical Society wasn't antiscience in the manner of Christian fundamentalists. Instead, it aimed at a synthesis of religion, science, and philosophy, a theory of everything rooted in the secret wisdom of the ancients. Mystical forces were to be investigated, understood, and mastered, just like physical principles. There was widespread optimism that even as traditional religion was losing its prestige, the scientific method could open supernatural realms to human comprehension. The young inventor Thomas Edison, a Theosophist who attended Blavatsky's salons, even dreamed of creating machines to test psychic powers and to communicate with the dead.

Theosophy ostensibly aimed to unite the essential truths underlying all religions, but the society (following Blavatsky herself) was always particularly interested in the East. As a child, Blavatsky had come into contact with the Kalmuck tribe, who lived on the Astrakhan steppes and practiced Tibetan Buddhism. Her grandfather was the Russian government's administrator for Kalmuck affairs, and her mother wrote a novel about the Kalmuck people. She almost certainly encountered Buddhist and Hindu teachers in her peripatetic thirties, and the Eastern element in her thinking grew more and more pronounced as time went on.

Blavatsky described herself as a Buddhist and claimed to be in communication with a pantheon of superhuman "Masters," Master Morya among them, who resided in the Himalayas. Letters from these Masters would materialize in Blavatsky's possession, though some of them displayed a remarkable taste for the kind of American slang that Madame herself enjoyed. Still, at least one sympathetic scholar, K. Paul Johnson, has argued that it's too simple to dismiss Blavatsky as merely a fraud. Instead, he argues, Blavatsky's "Masters" were mythologized versions of real teachers, including several reformers and revolutionaries. Indeed, Blavatsky maintained a mail correspondence with the Arya Samaj, a Hindu reform movement that sought to purge the religion of practices such as caste discrimination, child marriage, and idol worship.

In 1878, Blavatsky announced that she'd received orders from the Masters to move to India, and she and the ever-devoted Olcott promptly liquidated their possessions and set sail. It was a prescient decision: India was moving toward the center of the Western religious imagination and would soon become the preferred place of pilgrimage for Americans and Europeans seeking a transcendence they couldn't find in their own traditions. Yet, like all pioneers, Blavatsky and Olcott were also taking a big risk. As Washington writes, "They were reversing the usual flow of emigration from east to west, they were not young, and they had no capital to speak of."

After she moved to India, Blavatsky's fanciful accounts of subcontinental adventures were serialized in the Russian press. Madame Blavatsky, writes Sir Paul Dukes, "had many followers in her native land . . . Not a few there were who reveled in theories about other worlds because they fitted so ill into this one." One of them was Eugenia, who would later read everything by Blavatsky that she could get her hands on.

"The people at once had accepted her as one of their own," Eugenia would write decades later of Blavatsky's adventures in India. "They saw in her not a haughty foreigner but a loving friend." She told herself, "It will be the same when I go there."

Blavatsky wasn't the only major figure in Western esotericism to emerge from prerevolutionary Russia. Georges Ivanovich Gurdjieff, a mysterious, somewhat diabolical figure from the Caucasus with a self-created legend to rival Blavatsky's, had set himself up as a carpet dealer in Russia in 1912. Dukes met him while studying piano in St. Petersburg, before the start of Dukes's espionage career. Their first encounter was in Gurdjieff's modest apartment, decorated in his characteristic plush Orientalist style—intricate carpets, wrought-iron lamps, religious icons, *nargilah* (water pipes), and piles of multicolor cushions. Gurdjieff was thickset, with a bushy black beard and mischievous dark eyes, and wore a patterned silk dressing gown and a turban. He taught Dukes breathing techniques and the chanting of "Om," and soon they had become, in Dukes's words, *chela* and *guru*, or "student and master."

P. D. Ouspensky, then a journalist and a member of the St. Petersburg intelligentsia, met Gurdjieff in a Moscow café in 1915, not long after his own sojourn in India; he became Gurdjieff's pupil and, later, a famous occult philosopher in his own right. Rudolf Steiner, a brilliant Austrian whose movement, Anthroposophy, was a more Eurocentric spin-off of Theosophy, had an elite following in Russia's urban centers; the actor Michael Chekhov and the Russian poet and novelist Andrei Bely were both devotees (as was the man who would one day become Eugenia's second husband).

Yogic ideas, then, were part of a general mystical ferment during those last days of imperial Russia. Konstantin Balmont, one of the most important poets of the Silver Age, infused his work with Hindu notions and imagery, writing in the poem "Majja," "For the ignorant, life is delusion; for the yogi / It is illusion, a soulless ocean of silence!" Moscow's experimental Kamerny Theater opened at the end of 1914 with a performance of the Hindu classic drama *Shakuntala*, which Balmont translated from the Sanskrit.

For a dreamy, adventurous, artistic Russian girl, India could easily appear as a utopia—one that, as Blavatsky showed, a woman with enough daring could actually reach. Eugenia's fantasy India became a dream that would help her survive during the apocalypse that was soon upon her.

B Y THE SPRING of 1915, the front between Germany and Russia had reached Latvia. German troops would soon conquer the Latvian governorate of Courland. Worried that the Germans were about to march on Riga, Eugenia's grandmother, who had been born in St. Petersburg, decided to move the two of them to her native city, which had recently been renamed Petrograd so as to sound less German. Eugenia probably welcomed their flight: now she would be closer than ever to her mother.

Eugenia longed to follow her adored mother into a stage career. So, at sixteen, she enrolled in a school run by Claudia Isachenko, a former actress in Constantin Stanislavsky's Moscow Art Theater who, inspired by Isadora Duncan, had turned to modern dance. At the same time, Eugenia kept attending secondary school—her Riga school had relocated wholesale to Petrograd, so her education proceeded unbroken. She graduated with honors in 1916.

Life in Petrograd was at once giddy and hideous. It was the coldest winter in years. The war was going badly, and refugees were pouring into Russia's cities. Runaway inflation, coupled with the deterioration of the country's transportation system, created widespread food shortages in the city. "Everyone was affected: the industrial and white-collar workers and, in time, the lower ranks of the bureaucracy and even police employees," writes the historian Richard Pipes. Child prostitutes filled the streets. People slept outside food shops.

Among the rich, a kind of nihilistic gaiety prevailed. They binged on champagne and caviar, had heedless affairs, and threw away their fortunes in casinos. "We do not take defeat amiss, / And victory gives us no delight / The source of all our cares is this: / Can we get vodka for tonight?" went an anonymous poem written that year. Everyone else suffered, nurturing fears of imminent apocalypse or wild hopes of spiritual and political salvation.

By 1917, opposition to the decadent, callous, incompetent monarchy had become nearly universal, and in February, when a bread riot turned into the popular revolution that swept Russia's rulers from power, the ecstasy was widespread. Cafés threw open their doors for fellow citizens to feast for free. People kissed and even made love in the streets. In a letter to his mother, the poet Alexander Blok exulted, "A miracle has happened, and we may expect more miracles." There was an extraordinary feeling in the air, he writes, "that nothing is forbidden," that "almost anything might happen."

The crowds were volatile, ecstatic but also angry; the czar's hated police were a particular target of people's long-suppressed fury. Armed mobs attacked police stations and prisons, setting inmates free and often burning the buildings to the ground. Police records were torched in bonfires in the streets.

Eugenia grew up in a building owned by the police and surely understood that her beloved grandfather had been part of the system now being so deliriously destroyed. Yet she shared the thrill of February. "All of us who had dreams and projects," she writes, felt carried along "by the reviving spirit of those times." The last aristocratic constraints on her artistic ambitions had been swept away. Now nothing could stop her from becoming an actress like her mother.

When her grandmother went to join Sasha in Moscow, Eugenia quickly followed. There, to her delight, she was accepted at Theodore Komisarjevsky's theater school. Slight and intense, Komisarjevsky was an experimental director who set himself in opposition to Konstantin Stanislavsky, the Russian theater's most titanic figure. He rejected Stanislavsky's naturalism and his deeply psychological methods of creating characters, in favor of a far more stylized approach. Komisarjevsky's work was, if anything, emboldened by the revolution. In March 1917 he staged *On Alexis, Man of God*, a religious comedy by Mikhail Kuzmin, Russia's first openly gay writer, which had previously been banned by church censorship.

Komisarjevsky was a demanding teacher, impatient with students who failed to grasp his instruction. During an improvisation class, he barked at one of Eugenia's friends, "You twist like a rag doll and believe that is acting!" When it was Eugenia's turn, she was terrified. Terror, as it happened, was just what was called for—she had to improvise on the theme "the great scare," using only a table and chairs as props. Her scenario doesn't seem terribly inspired: she imagined herself dressing to go out, opening a door to look at herself in the mirror, and being frightened by a darting mouse. Screaming, she feigned panic as she climbed onto a table.

In a few moments, the maestro pronounced his verdict. Her improvisation was, he said, "more or less," his voice trailing off. That was it. At first, Eugenia was crushed, but her friends assured her that anything short of her teacher's all-out contempt was something to celebrate.

It pained Eugenia's grandmother to lose yet another family member to the stage, but she eventually resigned herself to her granddaughter's career, perhaps because it was the least of her worries. Russia's provisional government was weak, powerless to stop the strikes. Inflation and lawlessness paralyzed the country. There was anarchy in the streets, tempered only by ferocious outbursts of mob justice. Like everyone in the city, Eugenia waited on interminable lines for food and often returned home empty-handed.

In October, the Bolsheviks staged their coup. Armed fighting broke out in the streets of Moscow, the opening act of the Russian Civil War. For several days people were afraid to leave their houses, but even staying home could be dangerous: once, as Eugenia climbed the stairs inside her building, a stray bullet broke the window, whizzing by her head and into the wall beside her.

Like other aristocratic households, her family lost its fortune overnight. As a student, Eugenia was entitled to small rations of bread, oil, and sugar, which she shared with her grandmother, who finally had to admit that the young woman's acting career had some benefits.

For all the terror and volatility of those days, however, something in the unmoored atmosphere left Eugenia electrified. Forced for the first time in her life to be self-reliant, she was able to channel the idle anxiety of her childhood into action. She relished the freedom to go out at night on her own, attending theater premieres and hanging out at literary cafés, where she met futurist poets such as Vadim Shershenevich and Igor Severyanin, a decadent, flamboyantly cynical aesthete who always carried a lily in his hand.

Still, by the time Eugenia became Indra Devi, her habits of relentlessly positive thinking and her buoyant, ingenuous approach to life could, at times, obscure reality. There is very little darkness in her memoirs, even when she writes about the bleakest of times. People are constantly praising her, and even the most harrowing episodes have a magical way of working themselves out. While it's true that she had an astonishing ability to glide along the surface of earthshaking events, it's extremely unlikely that she escaped from the revolution entirely unscathed. All around her, the country was turning into hell—and she was learning a lesson that would serve her for the rest of her long life: how to survive her world's collapse by reinventing herself.

By the winter of 1918, writes Antony Beevor, "So many horses had been slaughtered for meat that carts and *drozhkys* were hauled by women and children." Members of the intelligentsia burned their books to stay warm. In the years to follow, writes Beevor, "[m]ost young actresses were forced to resort to part-time prostitution[,] and venereal disease was rife."

There's no evidence that Eugenia was forced to prostitute herself, but she must have suffered far more than she later let on. Komisarjevsky described some of what Moscow actors endured during the revolution in his 1929 book, *Myself and the Theatre:* "One morning when a young actress of my Theatre did not turn up to rehearsal we discovered that she had died of typhus during the night alone in a freezing room . . . A scenery designer suddenly and mysteriously disappeared, and we were told later that as a former Imperial officer and involved in some conspiracy he had been arrested and shot during the night by the Cheka [secret police]. One of the greatest character actresses in Russia, O. O. Sadovskaya, died of vermin."

Eugenia's mother had escaped Moscow's privations by going on tour, and she was soon living in Kiev, Ukraine, which had recently been seized by the Germans. In the summer of 1918, Eugenia decided to join her. Initially, she tried to get a permit at the German embassy in Moscow, but the disorderly crowd horrified her—she had a lifelong inability to deal with bureaucracy—so, she wrote, she traveled without one. She would later tell a story about this trip that, if true, is typical of her combination of audacity, recklessness, and excellent luck; her ability to remain untouched by calamity.

With a guide arranged by her mother, Eugenia made her way to the Ukrainian border, traveling partly on foot and partly in a packed, squalid third-class train car. Hunger tormented them, and her guide would read longingly from a cookbook he carried with him as if it were pornography.

In Ukraine, Eugenia boarded a Kiev-bound train. Soon, a German guard started making his way down the compartment, checking everyone's permits. For a moment, she didn't know what would happen when he reached her. Then she had an idea. She got up and walked, confidently and purposefully, into the cars that were reserved for German officers, sat down as if she belonged there, and pretended to be engrossed in a book. When the guard entered the carriage, he believed she was the girlfriend of someone important and marked her ticket without asking for her papers.

In Kiev, Eugenia joined her mother in a magnificent hotel, where food was in abundance. Teeming with refugees from the revolution, Kiev in the middle of 1918 "had an atmosphere of frenzied excitement, with everyone living as if there was no tomorrow," as the historian Orlando Figes writes. Mikhail Bulgakov describes the scene in his semiautobiographical novel, *The White Guard:*

> All spring . . . the City had been filling up with new arrivals.
> They slept in apartments on sofas and chairs. They dined in
> large companies at tables in luxurious apartments. Innumer-
> able shops opened selling comestibles and engaged in trade
> until late in the night, as did cafes where coffee was served
> and you could buy a woman, and there were new theaters . . .
> on whose boards increasingly famous actors who had fled the
> two capitals entertained and amused the public . . . [A]t night
> string music played in the cabarets . . . and faces of unearthly
> beauty shone on white, emaciated prostitutes hopped up on
> cocaine.

For all the scene's seediness, its familiarity must have been a terrific relief to Eugenia and Sasha. They stayed all summer and into the autumn, when Sasha got an acting job in another Ukrainian city, Kharkov, and Eugenia joined her. There, she befriended young poets and artists, including cabaret singer Alexander Vertinsky and the ravishing young actress Valentina Sanina. A star of prerevolutionary Moscow cabarets, Vertinsky was a slender, elegant man who powdered his face and darkened his eyes like a Russian Pierrot. He was famous for songs that mixed sorrowful melodrama with a louche touch of irony and exoticism; they had names such as "Cocaine Lady" and "Your Fingers Smell of Incense." Vertinsky was desperately in love with the enchanting, aloof Sanina, rhapsodizing in his memoirs about her "[e]normous, serene blue eyes with long lashes . . . a slim hand with long fingers of rare beauty." At his urging, he and Eugenia were constantly taking troikas, three-horse sleighs, to visit her. This friendship proved fortunate, for Sanina was to play a small but crucial role in Eugenia's later life.

The war caught up with Eugenia in 1919, when the Red Army took the city. For Eugenia, Sasha, and those of their theater colleagues who stayed behind, it would have been a terrifying time. Once again, food disappeared from the shelves. Kharkov's Chekists, or Bolshevik secret police, were known for plunging a victim's hand into boiling water and peeling the skin off like a glove. (Other Chekists devised tortures out of Eugenia's worst nightmares: they buried victims alive or interred them in coffins with corpses.) Despite the chaos and terror, though, some semblance of normal life seems to have continued, as it almost always does. There was still theater, which meant there was still work. A touring company from the legendary Moscow Art Theater even arrived in Kharkov in May, though performances began at 6:00 p.m. so guests could be home before the 9:00 p.m. curfew.

Sasha and her theater friends did their best to keep their spirits up. At night, they turned their depressing hotel rooms into little salons, reciting poetry and performing theatrical scenes by the dim light of a tiny lamp, acting as if they were still carefree artists in Moscow.

Eugenia, meanwhile, found work with a theater founded by the Moscow actor and director Vsevolod Alexandrovich Blumental-Tamarin, though apparently their relationship ended badly when she refused his advances. In a photo taken at that time, she's dressed in what looks like a low-cut nurse's costume, an exaggerated cross on a thick chain hanging around her neck. Her light brown curls are tucked into an oversize white cap. Rather than conventionally beautiful, Eugenia was what the French call *jolie laide*—striking from some angles and plain from others, with a slightly bulbous nose and a long chin. In that picture, though, as she gazes out with hooded, sultry eyes, she appears very much the ingénue.

Soon the city changed hands once again. The Moscow Art Theater was performing *The Cherry Orchard* when a commotion from the street interrupted the second act. Going outside, the stage manager learned that the forces of General Anton Denikin, head of the anti-Bolshevik White Army, were entering the city, and the Red Guards had fled. The audience broke into cheers, and the play resumed where it had left off.

The restaurants opened; once again there was food in abundance. "Where did all this come from?" Eugenia wondered with amazement.

The White Army was certainly no more humane than the Red; it was viciously anti-Semitic and implacably antidemocratic. Whenever it seized a town, soldiers were given a couple of days to plunder the property of local Jews. In a demented inversion of Bolshevik terror, some Whites shot workers just for being workers, their slogan, "Death to the Callused Hands!" echoing the Reds' "Death to the Burzhoois!"

Yet people such as Eugenia and Sasha, aristocratic and essentially apolitical, were safe behind White lines. When summer came, mother and daughter moved to Kislovodsk, a fashionable spa town in the Caucasus that the Whites had taken in January.

For Eugenia, Kislovodsk was "an enchanted corner" amid the squalor and terror of the war. She would take long walks through the surrounding forests and the city's public parks, while Sasha luxuriated in the town's thermal baths. One day, Eugenia returned from one of her walks to find a White Russian army officer in her hotel room. At first, she was startled and afraid. Then she recognized him. It was Vava Tretiakovy, her childhood playmate.

Vava had a guileless face, pleasing but largely nondescript, and gray eyes. His head was completely shaved. Eugenia found him to be devastatingly handsome. Her heart beat fast and her words came out awkwardly when she asked him, "What brings you here?"

"I came to see you," he replied.

It had been five years since they'd last met. Vava was now twenty-three and a lieutenant in the White Army. He'd contracted typhus—there was a raging epidemic of the lice-borne disease throughout the country—and had been sent to a sanitarium in Kislovodsk to recover. At first, they were shy and hesitant with each other, but eventually their old rapport returned, and soon they were joking and laughing. Then the conversation turned serious, and Vava told Eugenia he'd been pursuing a career as a composer when the war interrupted his studies. He'd also gotten married, though it was a loveless match, and he and his wife were close to separation.

Eugenia started taking her long walks with Vava. He spoke to her about all the death he'd seen and read her poems he'd written at the front, which she found captivating. As the summer went on, they admitted, to themselves and each other, that they were utterly in love. Acquaintances warned them not to spend so much time together, especially in public—he was, after all, still a married man. Eugenia, characteristically, didn't care. She had learned from her mother to ignore petty gossip and conventional opinion.

Their summer idyll, of course, soon came to an end. One day, as fall approached, Vava told his sweetheart he had to return to the war. They were sitting in the garden of Eugenia's boardinghouse. Eight decades later, she still remembered the small waterfall there and the green, moss-covered rocks beneath the water. Vava read her another poem he'd written for her, and she begged him, in vain, not to go.

They had three more days together, and they spent them returning again and again to the places they'd frequented during the summer, engraving them in their memories. On one of their walks, they ran into a photographer who made a living snapping vacationers. In the picture he took of them, they're sitting on the grass, leaning into each other. Vava is dressed in his uniform, while Eugenia wears a long, loose dress or skirt and high-heeled boots. Her smile is warm. His is faint and anxious.

His departure should have been the kind of scene later immortalized in countless war movies. She accompanied him to the station, which was full of people, anguished relatives bidding good-bye to soldiers trying to remain stoic. Tobacco smoke and the sound of women's sobbing filled the air. Eugenia must have prepared for a dramatic farewell, to wave at her love until the train disappeared.

Yet the train never came, and Vava walked her home. "See you soon, my little girl," he said on the threshold to her house. The next morning, when she went to find him, he'd already left.

They wrote each other regularly, letters that were passionate and fervidly romantic, almost religious in their youthful ecstasy. At one point, Eugenia decided to travel to the front herself to see her lover, but he begged her not to come, saying it was too dangerous.

Already the war's privations were coming to serene Kislovodsk. Eugenia traded most of her remaining clothes and jewelry for food. Her mother had already left town for another job. Eugenia headed to Pyatigorsk, a city in the Caucasus where an old friend was living. Once again, she found work in the theater.

Vava's letters, once so regular, stopped arriving, and she waited in a panic as months went by. Then five came at once, and she could see his despair building from one to the next. First, he hoped he'd soon be transferred to a town where they could meet. Then he started fearing they'd never see each other again. He felt desperately alone in the army; another soldier had struck him, and Vava's failure to avenge himself had left him humiliated. He was even considering deserting. Eugenia wrote to console him, but she never heard back.

By the spring of 1920, the White Army was almost completely defeated, and those who survived fled to Paris, Berlin, or Constantinople. Eugenia wrote to officials in all those countries, seeing if any knew of a Lieutenant Tretiakovy. The absence of any news about Vava tormented her. She worried that he had fallen in one of the final battles, or even committed suicide, though she also nurtured fantasies that he'd escaped to the other side of the world, "for example to Patagonia," a destination that, she wrote, had fascinated him.

She would never see or hear from him again.

That line about Patagonia is her first and only mention of Vava's love of the wild desert region stretching across Chile and Argentina. She doesn't tell us why her lover dreamed of South America, but the memory seems significant, since she would start a new life there more than sixty years later.

Eugenia had lost contact with her mother. At one point, she thought Sasha had joined the White Russian exodus to Constantinople. More than one hundred thousand Russians had fled there along with the

White Russian general Pyotr Nikolayevich Wrangel, and the city was full of Russian theaters, clubs, and restaurants where aristocratic Russian women waited table.

Yet a friend who'd recently been in that city assured Eugenia that her mother wasn't there, so Eugenia set off through the cities of Russia and the Caucasus searching for her, refusing to entertain the thought that she might be dead. These trips, which would have been taken in filthy, crowded third-class trains, amid a wrathful peasantry eager for revenge against the upper classes and the ever-present threat of arbitrary arrest, were probably harrowing. Her account of them, though, has a picaresque tone, as she eludes danger time and again.

One day, she was pulled off a train en route from Tiflis. This is how she recalls the conversation with her interrogator, a Russian military policeman:

"Were you in Tiflis?"

"Yes," she answered.

"What were they doing there?"

"Who? Everyone?" she replied mockingly. "Some are newspaper sellers, others work in the restaurants, and others are actors and actresses, like me."

Such insolence could have gotten her killed. Instead, as she tells it, the guard took her to a house where she could stay overnight. She thought he was going to protect her, but in the middle of the night, there was a pounding on her door. "Police! Open the door!" came their shouts. It was the Cheka. Eugenia had the presence of mind to hide Vava's letters between a picture and its frame—had the secret police found them and realized she was the girlfriend of a White soldier, she'd have been executed. Instead, she was merely arrested.

Her memoirs suggest that she spent only a few days in jail, but it was probably quite a bit longer. Upon coming to the United States in 1947, she had to report any imprisonments on an INS form. On it, she said she'd been held for a month, and a few years after that, she told an INS agent that it had been a couple of weeks. Devi, unlike most modern memoirists, tended to play down her own misfortunes, casting a rosy, magical glow around her history. She could never afford to dwell on trauma, and eventually she made letting go of the past the centerpiece of her personal spirituality.

After being released, as she told the story, she went back to the house where she'd been arrested to get Vava's letters. There she found the military policeman who'd betrayed her, and she bitterly reproached him about her unjust imprisonment. Then, right in front of him, she took the letters from their hiding place. "If you want to arrest me, you can do it now, this instant," she exclaimed.

"You must burn those immediately!" he shouted.

"I wouldn't do it for anything in the world!" she said triumphantly, pressing them against her chest.

There's no way, of course, to confirm that this anecdote is true. It may well be simply what she wished had happened. Indisputably true, though, is the way Eugenia would make an aura of invulnerability a cornerstone of her persona.

From there, Eugenia traveled back to Kislovodsk. Then she heard, likely from someone else in the theater, that her mother was in Odessa, so she traveled to that city. By the time she arrived, Sasha had moved on.

Months passed before she finally tracked her mother down to a town on the Russian-Polish border. Sasha was thin, her clothes worn, and she was living in a modest, spartanly furnished room. She had hooked up with a dozen other Russian actors, and they eked out a living performing in the small cities and towns nearby, while making plans to flee Russia. Eugenia joined them, devoting herself to plans of escape.

By this time, Latvia had declared its independence, commencing two decades as a sovereign republic. Eugenia's grandmother had returned to Riga. Technically, Eugenia and Sasha should have been able to get Latvian passports and leave Russia legally. Yet Eugenia felt paralyzed by the almost Kafkaesque process that getting such papers would entail. Sneaking over the border into Poland seemed more straightforward.

The region of Russia where they were living was separated from Poland by a river, which was then frozen. Eugenia, her mother, and her mother's friends paid two men to help them across.

On the night they left, each took only what he or she could carry in a small bag and walked to an appointed place near the river at the city's edge. Banks of snow almost hid the river's frozen surface from view. They were told to run as fast as they could when they heard a whistle. One sounded, and they took off. The Russian guards had been bribed, and rather than shooting at the fleeing party, they shot into the air. In a few minutes, the actors arrived in Poland. There, the Polish authorities quickly arrested them.

They were brought to what Eugenia recalled as a stately house that had been transformed into a prison. Being with Sasha made imprisonment an entirely different experience—having craved closeness with her mother all her life, Eugenia was thrilled that they could finally have long, unbroken conversations. Along with the actors, there were common criminals in the prison, who tried to comfort the new arrivals, even promising to come back and rescue them if they were set free first. "Smiling to myself," Devi writes, "I thought, 'Look who are my best friends: bandits!'"

Soon the actors were released, and they started performing again, in the small cities along the border, finding an audience among the Russian landowners who lived in Poland. Yet, if life improved, Eugenia was still desperate in her search for Vava. She continued sending out an endless stream of letters, all of them disappearing into the ether. At night, she reread his letters and poems, or compulsively copied them in her own hand. She grew morbid and would spend hours alone in the small chapel of a nearby cemetery.

Further, after having chased her mother for so many years, Eugenia now found she disliked performing with her mother's group. She longed to do real theater instead of gaudy, improvised entertainments and wondered what would ever become of the great plans and ambitions she'd nurtured through her adolescence. In her diary, she wrote that she felt weighed down as if by a bag of stones.

In this sad, unsettled new life, Eugenia turned to an old fantasy to sustain her: India. The dream that had been born when she encountered Ramacharaka's book all those years ago had never left her. Amid the chaos and ugliness all around her, she writes, "India appeared to me as a country that was fresh, colorful and beautiful."

Yet that escape would come later. Throughout 1922, Eugenia and Sasha had made endless, seemingly futile trips to Polish government offices, trying to get papers that would allow them to move abroad. Finally, toward the end of the year, they succeeded—thanks, Eugenia writes, to a bureaucrat who was a devoted fan of a Russian singer whom Sasha knew.

So, in 1923, Eugenia and Sasha arrived together in Berlin, the dazzling, depraved, and intrigue-filled capital of the White Russian emigration. It was the year that lunatic inflation erased the savings of the German middle class and Hitler staged his famous Beer Hall Putsch in Munich. Yet Berlin was madly festive, perhaps the most artistically vibrant city in the world, and for a while, Eugenia would revel in it.

AS THE WHITE ARMY collapsed in Russia, unmoored Russians streamed into Berlin in one of the largest mass emigrations of modern times. They arrived in a city that was already growing explosively: Berlin's population had doubled from two million in 1905 to four million in 1920, and the Russians added another half million. So many Russians settled in Charlottenburg, a once-fashionable neighborhood in western Berlin, that it became known as Charlottengrad, and the Kurfürstendamm, the boulevard bordering the neighborhood, was dubbed the Nevsky Prospekt, after the main street in St. Petersburg.

"After the war, Berlin had become a kind of caravansary where everyone traveling between Moscow and the West came together," Marc Chagall would recall years later. "In the apartments round the Bayrische Platz [*sic*] there were as many samovars and Theosophical and Tolstoyan countesses as there had been in Moscow . . . in my whole life I've never seen so many wonderful rabbis or so many Constructivists as in Berlin in 1922." Russian restaurants lined the streets. There were three Russian newspapers, five weekly magazines, and an endless profusion of publishing houses.

Eugenia and Sasha quickly made themselves at home in Berlin's

Russian colony. They found rooms in Charlottenburg, and were soon reuniting with friends they'd lost track of during the revolution and civil war. Sasha found work with one of Berlin's Russian theaters, while Eugenia gloried in the city's febrile artistic atmosphere, its heady mix of innovation, insecurity, decadence, and mysticism.

At the time, Berlin was the most modern city in Europe, a gritty, jittery metropolis given to both extravagant cynicism and desperate grabs at redemption. Germany's defeat in World War I had led to the abdication of the Kaiser and the birth of a weak, unstable liberal democracy. The economy had been savaged by the war, and as the government borrowed and printed money to pay its war debts, hyperinflation destroyed both the German mark and the whole country's sense of material security. In July 1922 the dollar was worth 493 marks. By March of 1923, a dollar bought more than 20,000 marks, and by the end of the year, it was worth a ludicrous 4.2 trillion marks.

The berserk inflation made hard assets paramount, and Russians who'd smuggled jewels out of their country could often live comfortably by peddling the ornaments of their vanished privilege. "Herds of foreigners wandered along the Kurfürstendamm: they were buying up the remnants of former luxury for a song," wrote Ilya Ehrenburg, the Russian author and journalist.

For ordinary Germans, though, inflation meant financial calamity. The middle class found its savings wiped out overnight, even as a few speculators became fantastically rich. A great many women were forced into the sex trade: by the mid-1920s, there were around one hundred thousand prostitutes in Berlin, ten times as many as in present-day Amsterdam. Whatever money people had, they wanted to spend as quickly as possible, before it lost value. An orgy of consumption commenced amid crushing poverty. Because it was impossible to save for the future, everyone was forced to live in the garish, whirling present.

Many people expected imminent Communist revolution—some with dread, some with thrilling hope. Right-wing paramilitary groups operated with impunity, often receiving support from White Russians whose loathing of Bolshevism burned with religious intensity. Between 1918 and 1922, there were nearly four hundred political murders, the vast majority committed by reactionaries, who targeted leftists and moderate leaders alike. "The indifference with which one greets political murders and the victims of turbulent street demonstrations today in Germany is to be explained by the fact that the war has numbed us to the value of human life," despaired the economist Emil Julius Gumbel.

Amid the economic and political chaos, Berliners sought relief in frantic, end-of-the-world binges of sex, drugs, and dancing. There was a mania for jazz, the music of anarchic modernity. Jazz "unifies within itself everything that remains from the great collapse of the world and humanity, dances with it over the abyss," wrote one critic.

The end of the *Kaiserreich* meant the end of most forms of censorship, so all over the city, seedy variety shows featured rows of naked women. The cabaret number "Take It Off, Petronella!" satirized the craze for stripping: "Of your talent we're adoring / But we find the theater boring / If you don't want us to yawn or snore or cough / Take it off, Petronella, take it off!" The proto-performance artist Anita Berber presented her dark, wild expressionistic dances naked or nearly so on Berlin's cabaret stages, sometimes appearing bound by ropes in sadomasochistic duets with her openly gay second husband, Sebastian Droste. In her off-hours, she hung out in nightclubs and casinos, often dressed in nothing but a sable wrap, heels, and a silver brooch packed with cocaine.

The flip side of this aggressive dissoluteness was a widespread longing for purity and divinity. Given Eugenia's interest in esoteric religion, she must have enjoyed Berlin's vast buffet of alternative spirituality. In Russia, dabbling in the occult was limited mostly to elites. In Weimar Germany, it was a mass phenomenon. An anxious representative of the Catholic Church noted in 1923 that more than ten thousand families in Munich alone had held séances. Police departments all over the country hired clairvoyants for help in solving crimes. Hypnotists and stage magicians often wrapped themselves in Eastern religious garb. Some Jewish occults claimed Indian heritage "and swore on their mezuzahs that they were Brahmins," in the words of historian Mel Gordon.

There was enormous interest in yoga and other Indian religious practices. "Aspiring occultists who . . . studied with the Berlin magnetist and Theosophical publisher Paul Zillmann learned to maintain purity of both spirit and flesh by opening their day with a snort of cold water through the nose, doing their occult exercises while taking deep breaths of fresh air, and sharply limiting their intake of such spirit-disturbing substances as alcohol, strong spices, and caffeinated drinks," writes historian Corinna Treitel. Much of this will sound familiar to hatha yoga practitioners: Snorting water to clean out the sinuses is a well-known *kriya*, or cleansing practice, and exercises coupled with deep breathing are known as asanas. Many yoga teachers recommend what's called a *sattvic* diet, which abjures not just intoxicants but strong spices as well.

Germany's fascination with magic and Eastern religion combined with the indigenous craze for *Lebensreform*, or "life reform," a sort of countercultural back-to-nature reaction to modern urban life. *Lebensreform* emphasized bodily purity through diet, rhythmic gymnastics, homeopathic medicine, nudism, and communion with nature. It was deeply mystical—writing in 1927, the critic Wolfgang Graeser celebrated the development of "new, influential metaphysics" based on self-discovery and "a search for physical and spiritual unity."

Both *Lebensreform* and German occultism more generally would branch out in terrifyingly reactionary directions. Nazi ideology, with its obsession with bodily health and purity, appropriation of Hindu symbols, and faith in the mystical destiny of the Aryan race, incorporated elements of the two movements. Indeed, even though Theosophy championed the worldwide brotherhood of man, in Germany and Austria a racist spin-off called Ariosophy developed. Ariosophy borrowed Theosophy's cosmology but turned its morality upside down, and it ended up playing a small but important role in the advent of Nazism. As Treitel points out, it was an Ariosophical circle that hosted the meeting during which the Deutsche Arbeiterpartei (German Workers' Party), the predecessor to the Nazi Party, was founded.

Yet *Lebensreform* wasn't inherently reactionary: politically, its adherents, like those of the occult milieu more generally, were all over the map. "[A]gainst every instance of *völkisch* or Nazi enthusiasm for alternative medicine, including occult medicine, one could proffer a counterexample," writes Treitel. She cites the healer Alexander Müller, whose book *Cosmic and Earthly Rays as Disease Pathogens* ends with a call for human unity to triumph over racist nationalism. More often still, *Lebensreform* and occultism were simply apolitical, promising personal salvation rather than systemic change.

Ultimately *Lebensreform*, which saw the cultivation of a healthy body as the road to spirituality and self-realization, prefigured modern yoga culture in the West. It would have an obvious influence on the future Indra Devi. Yet, at the moment, Eugenia was less concerned with transcendence than with artistic exploration. Eager to establish her identity as an actress, she was naturally drawn to the city's scintillating cabarets.

Cabaret, of course, was the prototypical art form of Weimar Berlin. Though *Cabaret*, the Broadway musical and film that immortalized the genre, is set during the rise of Nazism, Berlin cabaret actually peaked in the early 1920s. Miniature festivals of urbane nihilism, the cabarets were customarily held in small, intimate theaters, where guests could drink champagne and dine. Usually a smooth, tuxedoed *conférencier* presided over the show, which consisted of songs and sketches that knowingly eviscerated the city's fashions, its mania for sex and film stars, and its politics.

In one Dadaist cabaret, grotesque puppets created by the painter George Grosz imitated stars of the political scene. One representing Kurt Eisner, the socialist prime minister of Bavaria who'd been assassinated in 1919, offered a bitter monologue: "The whole thing's lost every trace of romance, / The hero's pose, the stately stance. / There's no more crown and no more throne, / In short, it's just not worth a bone."

Dirnenlieder, or whores' songs, were a cabaret staple. At once titillating and sentimental, they often began with a woman standing in a pool of red light and announcing, "Ich bin eine Dirne" ("I am a whore"). She'd recount her miseries and degradations in song, all for the delectation of stylish audiences who'd come to fetishize their city's criminal underworld.

In this caustic, numbing atmosphere, the Russian cabaret Der Blaue Vogel was an oasis of sweetness and delicacy. Opening in 1921, it became a Berlin sensation precisely because it was so different from most of what made Berlin sensational.

Der Blaue Vogel—the name means "the Bluebird" in German—was a colorful, elaborate fairy-tale spectacle, a children's book come to life, though with a touch of winking adult irony. The company's founder, Jascha Jushny, had occasionally performed as the *conférencier* at the Bat, a prerevolutionary cabaret in Moscow, and he drew on his experiences there for his new venture. Yet techniques that had seemed avant-garde in pre–World War I Russia—actors rebelling against naturalism by impersonating mechanical dolls; songs and sketches that drew on the colorful primitivism of Russian folk culture—seemed magically quaint in postwar Berlin.

Der Blaue Vogel appealed both to the pained nostalgia of the émigrés and to the locals' lust for novelty. Sets featured elaborate, riotously colorful, and graphically extravagant backdrops by leading theater artists who blended Art Nouveau, Cubist, and Constructivist influences. The shows were playfully surreal, with heads popping out of furniture to sing, or toys coming suddenly to life. Sometimes actors were positioned behind paintings with life-size cutouts, so that the murals seemed to talk. There were numbers based on old Russian legends and on life in czarist Russia, and more modern sketches such as "Time Is Money," about the hectic mechanized rush of modern society. Somehow, it was all imbued with a sense of ethereal naïveté, a deliberate innocence.

One critic called Der Blaue Vogel a "pearl of the light genre . . . On seeing these things, one swears by cubism. Here the pattern fits. It produces modernism of a fairy-tale-like pithiness—irresistible." Another described it as "a world, glowing in colours, animated with creatures, gigantic or dwarfish, full of music, bizarre ideas, fun improbability and surprise." The poet Else Lasker-Schüler, a well-known figure in avant-garde circles, enthused, "Der Blaue Vogel is the most wonderful thing here in the world one can see."

Naturally, Eugenia had to experience the cabaret that all Berlin was talking about. And when she did, she was enchanted. She felt its spirit "completely in tune with my own," at once whimsical and sophisticated, avant-garde and innocent. She was determined to become part of it.

Joining Der Blaue Vogel, however, wasn't easy. Places in the cast were much sought after, and besides, there weren't any openings. Before long, though, Eugenia learned that Jushny was assembling a touring company. She auditioned and, thrillingly, was cast. It was, for her, an incandescent moment. After the miseries and terrible dislocations of the war, life was opening up in front of her. She had finally emerged from her mother's shadow, becoming an actress in her own right.

Soon her happiness was compounded when, after years of mourning Vava, Eugenia fell in love again. The object of her affection was Fryderyk Járosy, an aristocratic ex-journalist who wrote songs and sketches for Der Blaue Vogel and served as *conférencier* when Jushny was absent. "When I met him, I felt the storm clouds obscuring my life lift," she writes.

It's easy to see why she was smitten—most people who met Járosy were. Ten years older than Eugenia, he had fine, elegant features; an ironic gleam in his dark eyes; and impeccable manners. He spoke five languages fluently. Back in Moscow, the famous Russian actor Michael Chekhov, Anton Chekhov's nephew, had found Járosy impressive even though he was sleeping with Chekhov's wife. "He was an adventurer of the sort about which my father had recounted many fascinating stories," Chekhov writes. "Elegant, good-looking, charming and talented as he was, he had at his disposal a great inner strength, which made him irresistible."

Járosy was born in Prague, son of a half-Hungarian, half-Croat father and an Austrian mother. He married into an aristocratic Russian family—he met his wife, Natalia, at the Swiss sanitarium that served as the inspiration for Thomas Mann's *The Magic Mountain*. The two seem to have been separated in the chaos following the Russian Revolution, when Járosy became involved with the ravishing young Olga Chekhova.

At the time, Olga was trapped in a miserable marriage to Michael Chekhov, a celebrated actor but an unstable alcoholic who was tumbling into a nervous breakdown. He couldn't take care of Olga when the revolution came, and she wasn't used to taking care of herself.

Járosy, evidently, stepped in to help, his ironic sangfroid a tremendous comfort. "It was a period during which battles were still being fought on the Moscow streets, artillery shells exploded in the distance and bullets whistled past people's houses, often shattering their windows," writes Michael Chekhov's biographer, Charles Marowitz. "But Jaroszi, who came courting Olga, blithely walked the streets, visiting the family daily, imperturbable and consistently entertaining. He claimed that he couldn't be killed. 'If you can hold your life in contempt completely,' he said, 'then it is out of danger.'"

In 1920, Járosy helped Olga formulate a plan to escape from Moscow. According to her account, she dressed like a peasant woman, with a head scarf, felt boots, and a bulky overcoat, and took a train from Moscow's Belorussky Station with a diamond ring hidden under her tongue. Soon after arriving in Berlin, she threw Járosy over and went on to have an extraordinary career in European cinema, working with directors including F. W. Murnau, Alfred Hitchcock, and Max Ophüls. (During the Nazi years, she became a favorite of Adolf Hitler and Joseph Goebbels—the latter's diaries refer to her as "eine charmante Frau" [a charming woman]—all while working as a Soviet spy, though the extent of her intelligence activities remains something of a mystery.)

Járosy, meanwhile, found work in a publishing house and began writing newspaper articles, and numbers for Russian theaters. By 1921 he was part of Der Blaue Vogel. In an essay for the theater's first program, he described how the troupe was rooted in the Russian experience: "Tired of politics and everyday life, the Russian sought in his cabaret visit a complete release of the reality of life. He looked for merry self-abandonment in music, color, and playfulness ... Whether it was the production of a Chekhov humoresque, the stylization of everyday phenomenon [sic], the parody of an artistic genre, the dramatization of a chanson—it was always a close cooperation between the painter, musician, actor, director, and the muse of good taste."

Eugenia's affair with Járosy, whom she called by his middle name, Miroslav, unfolded in many of the great cities of Europe, as they traveled to perform in Geneva, Madrid, Prague, Budapest, and Vienna. The actors weren't paid much, but they were put up in grand hotels, and Eugenia developed close friendships while on tour. Almost everywhere they went, the reception was rapturous, which surely helped morale. The Berlin critic Ferdinand Hager, who followed foreign newspaper coverage of Der Blaue Vogel's tour, wrote, "[E]verywhere I read of victories, triumphs and cheers."

As long as Járosy was with her, Eugenia was ecstatic, but her dependence on him also became debilitating. One time, he was supposed to meet her and the rest of the troupe in Vienna. In her diary, she rhapsodized about the city's old backstreets and grand avenues, its ancient churches and sweet air free of the choking industrial exhaust of Berlin. She felt wonderful, attuned to the world's "sublime harmonies." Then word came that Járosy was ill and couldn't come as promised. Suddenly, she was shattered. Feeling as if she were going crazy, she shut herself up in her hotel room sobbing, terrified that he was lost to her.

That night, she was playing the role of Katenka, a mechanical Russian toy come to life. Onstage, anxiety overwhelmed her, and she froze. After a few minutes, she was able to complete the scene, but with difficulty. The audience, feeling defrauded, barely applauded.

She didn't begin to shine until Járosy finally showed up. Once he arrived, she was again exuberant, her acting rejuvenated. The next time she played Katenka, she received fulsome applause. Later, in Zurich, she and Járosy took long walks in the nearby forests and meadows, surrounded by the Alps. In an almost mystical state of romantic bliss, she felt as if the violets were smiling at her.

Her attachment to Járosy, though, would soon derail her career. In 1924 they were performing in Warsaw to enormous acclaim. Eugenia, said one reviewer, "captivated" the audience. The crowds adored Járosy—so much so that when Jushny arrived in town, he was irritated and more than a little jealous. According to several reports, Jushny pushed Járosy aside to become *conférencier* himself. Yet Polish audiences didn't take to Jushny and demanded the return of their favorite. This sparked a row between the two men, which ended with Járosy being fired.

Naturally, Eugenia took her lover's side and remonstrated with Jushny. He responded by firing her as well: At first, the sudden expulsion from what had become a kind of surrogate family left her stunned. After a couple of days, Jushny reconsidered and sent an assistant to try to persuade Eugenia to stay after all. By then, however, she'd decided that her time with Der Blaue Vogel, one of the happiest periods of her life, was finished. "The only thing that remained was the love of Miroslav," she writes.

Yet even that was far from secure. Járosy treated his lovers with exquisite tenderness, but not fidelity. Indeed, though Eugenia didn't know it, while in Warsaw he'd already begun an affair with the burgeoning Polish starlet Hanka Ordonówa, and soon the two were living together.

After leaving Der Blaue Vogel, Eugenia decided to visit her mother, who had recently returned to Riga, and to apply for a Latvian passport, which would allow her to travel more easily than her provisional German papers did. So, in the summer of 1924, she went back to the city of her birth. There, she performed in some of the same cabarets as Sasha—both of them were on the bill for a New Year's Eve celebration at something called the A.T. Café, which also featured actors from Riga's celebrated Russian Drama Theatre, and an American jazz band that performed with kitchen utensils. Early the next year, Eugenia and Sasha formed their own theater company, which premiered at the end of March, though it appears to have been short-lived.

Járosy sent her postcards from Paris, where he was looking for work, but once again the separation tormented Eugenia. Finally, at the start of 1925, he came to visit her. He was much changed—Eugenia thought the struggle to survive in the theater had worn him down. Nevertheless, they rekindled their affair, and her misery subsided, though when he left in February, it quickly returned. She had nightmares. Daily life was full of dark, even occult presentiments. Once, she found a brooch he'd given her on the floor; picking it up, she saw that it was cracked. Suddenly she was shot through with terror, convinced that this was an omen and that something unspeakable had happened to her love.

She suffered through the winter, but when spring came she was able to reunite with Járosy in Austria, and she hoped they'd be able to spend the summer together. They had a few lovely days, taking long walks through the mountains and eating picnics of cheese and fruit. Yet he was distant; she thought he was depressed. Then, he ended their relationship.

He told her, kindly, that he didn't want to be a burden to her and that she needed to discover her own path. She should go to India, he said, just as she'd always longed to. His words pierced her. Once again, her dreams of her future were being ripped away, but she realized she had no choice but to let him go.

It would be almost thirty years before they saw each other again.

By the time they parted, Járosy had moved permanently to Warsaw, where he'd been so warmly received when he was with Der Blaue Vogel. He became the emcee at Quid Pro Quo, the city's premier cabaret. "All of Warsaw's best comics, dancers, singers, and actors eventually appeared on the club's tiny stage," writes cabaret historian Ron Nowicki. Járosy couldn't speak Polish properly, but that just endeared him to the crowds all the more. He intoned "Proszę Państwa!" ("Ladies and gentleman!") with such grandeur that it became a popular catchphrase in sophisticated circles. Soon the new king of Warsaw cabaret accepted Polish citizenship.

On August 23, 1939, Germany and the Soviet Union signed the Molotov-Ribbentrop Pact, a nonaggression treaty. One week later, the two countries, along with the German client state of Slovakia, invaded Poland and divided it between themselves. Warsaw came under Nazi occupation. Járosy was outspoken in his hatred of the regime. He composed satirical anti-Nazi poems and scattered them all around the city. Sometimes he'd translate them into German and put them on German cars.

One began with this quote from a German newspaper: "The world's leading scholars have confirmed that the German is the epitome of the Nordic race." Járosy then wrote:

> Take Hitler's dark hair,
> and Goering's fat belly,
> and Goebbels' short height.
> Mix all this up a trace.
> What will come out of all that brown mess?
> The epitome of the Nordic race!

On October 25, 1939, Járosy was arrested by the Gestapo. At first the Nazis seemed more interested in co-opting the famous performer than in persecuting him. They offered him the chance to claim his *Reichsdeutsche* citizenship—he'd been Austrian, after all—and to run a German propaganda theater. Járosy refused. He was tried and convicted in March 1940, and sentenced to execution. Then, somehow, as he was being transported back to prison, he escaped. He spent the next four years in hiding in and around Warsaw.

Germany invaded the Soviet Union in 1941, pushing the latter to join the Allies. By the summer of 1944, the Polish resistance expected the imminent arrival of Soviet forces in Warsaw, and the former launched a rebellion to dislodge the Nazis. It was only intended to last for a few days, but the Soviets halted their advance, and the Poles had to fight alone. Járosy was among them, and the Nazis captured him.

On August 14 the Germans brought Járosy to Buchenwald. There, some higher-ranking Polish prisoners recognized him as a celebrated actor and brought him into their quarters, protecting him from the worst of the concentration camp's brutality.

The artist and poet Mieczysław Lurczyński met Járosy in one of Buchenwald's subcamps, and he became the inspiration for the character of Fryderyk in Lurczyński's searing play, *The Old Guard*. Lurczyński remembered Járosy as an icon of humanism and civilization amid the camp's savagery. "A conversation with him was an escape," he writes in his memoirs. "[I]t allowed me to get a breather from the primitiveness and bestiality surrounding me on all sides."

In the play, Fryderyk is tormented by the moral compromises that survival in the camp requires. The Polish prisoners who manage internal camp affairs are callous and vicious to the inmates over whom they rule, and Fryderyk hates his dependence on them. "Do you know that in here they consider me a non-kosher clown, who has to kow-tow and re-tell farces and risqué anecdotes under the threat of losing the favor of his lordship who knows that this stinking room is a palace compared to the hell of life in the barracks?" he says. Eventually he stands up to one of his protectors, threatening to denounce him when the war ends, to make sure he's held responsible for his cruelty. Fryderyk's desperate assertion of his obliterated society's values leads to his death.

In real life, however, Járosy didn't die. The camp was evacuated in March 1945, and the inmates were loaded onto an open-wagon train. When Allied strafing stalled it, Járosy and Lurczyński escaped. Járosy eventually made his way to London and spent the rest of his life performing for the Polish diaspora.

In the early 1950s he visited Los Angeles on tour. It's not clear how he and Indra Devi learned that they were once again in the same city, but each of them was thrilled and amazed to find the other still alive. After their reunion, Járosy, ever suave, wrote her a letter full of endearments. He recalled their beautiful times together and told her that he felt suddenly twenty years younger. They met again in 1960, when Devi stopped in London on the way home from a trip to Russia. Járosy told her she was the only woman he'd ever loved. That's almost certainly not true, but he probably said it as if he meant it.

Back in Riga in 1926, her liaison with Járosy over, Eugenia had nothing but work for consolation, so she threw herself back into acting, signing a contract with a Riga theater that styled itself after Der Blaue Vogel. There, she had the chance to do some directing, which she found enormously stimulating.

New suitors quickly came calling, though none of them was nearly as dashing or fascinating as Járosy. A former naval officer proposed to her, but convinced they had nothing in common, she turned him down. A German banker, Hermann Bolm, also began to frequent her house. Twenty years Eugenia's senior, he was married, though his wife had abandoned him and asked for a divorce. Eugenia found him charming, kind, and attractive. With his wavy black hair and olive skin, he seemed to her more Italian than German. In a photo from that time, she's sitting next to a girlfriend, smiling in a sequined flapper dress and Mary Jane heels. A shiny headband holds back her bobbed hair. He's behind her in a tuxedo and white tie, solid and protective.

She was twenty-seven, and it was unlikely that acting was ever going to earn her much of a living. She liked Bolm and believed she could be happy with him. It wasn't a great love, but given her precarious circumstances, it would do. So when his divorce was finalized and he asked her to marry him, she said yes.

From the start of their engagement, though, she was anxious. Her fiancé was kind but also controlling. He insisted that once they were married, she should leave the theater altogether, warning her, "When we're married, you will be totally under my control." His words chilled her. She had always valued her liberty above all else.

That summer, she traveled to Tallinn, the capital of Estonia, where her mother was performing. One day, she wandered into a bookstore advertising Theosophical literature. As she paged through the volumes, an employee handed her a flyer for an upcoming gathering of something called the Order of the Star in the East in Ommen, Holland. The order was devoted to heralding the teachings of a young Indian man named Jiddu Krishnamurti, believed by a group of leading Theosophists to be a new messiah. Thousands of people would be camping out on the grounds of a Dutch castle to hear Krishnamurti and his "protectress," Annie Besant, who had succeeded Madame Blavatsky as Theosophy's figurehead.

The group's name—full, she thought, of beauty and mystery—made an immediate impact on Eugenia. She wondered if perhaps her own star might be guiding her to discover the strange city of Ommen.

If she saw the flyer as a sign, it might have been because she was desperately seeking one. She was close to packing away her youthful dreams of India and settling down to a comfortable but compromised life as a bourgeois housewife. The Order of the Star in the East would have appeared as a last shot at transcendence. It wasn't India, but at the moment it was as close as Eugenia could get. When she returned to Riga, she went to the local Theosophical Society headquarters and registered for the Star meeting. And at the end of July, she boarded a train for Holland.

RRIVING IN Ommen, Holland, at the end of July 1926, Eugenia joined pilgrims from every corner of Europe and from the United States. There were at least two thousand of them, mostly aristocrats, bohemians, and intellectuals, but also proper middle-class housewives, and poor mystics who came on foot. Extra ferries from the British Isles to the Hook of Holland had to be scheduled to accommodate them all.

The writer Rom Landau's description of the crowd at the 1927 Star Camp would have been equally apt in 1926. "Such readers as have ever attended a theosophical or practically any sort of religious convention will know the type, and I shall refrain from describing it at length," he writes. "They generally abhor the idea of meat as violently as that of wine or tobacco; they look deep into your eyes when they talk to you; they have a weakness for sandals, for clothes without any particular distinction of shape, for the rougher kind of textiles and such colours as mauve, bottle-green and purple. The men affect long hair, while the women keep theirs short."

The Order of the Star gathering took place on the forested grounds of Eerde Castle, which was donated to the order by a Dutch aristocrat named Baron Philip van Pallandt. Important people in the Star organization stayed in the castle itself, an eighteenth-century Dutch classical building ringed by a moat, with pavilions on each side. A formal circular garden fronted the building, which was surrounded by parkland where most of the attendees slept in small canvas tents.

An Associated Press dispatch about the event carried the lurid headline "Secrecy Veils Cult Camp," but the piece painted a pleasant, bucolic picture. "The camp is beautifully situated on the slopes of Best-Hnerberg [*sic*], its multicolored and multishaped tents dominated by two giant ones set apart for meetings and meals. These can be seen for miles, surmounted by Dutch and American flags," it read. "The tents are arranged in pleasing disorder, some labeled 'married,' others 'ladies' and others 'gentlemen,' all trim and comfortable." In some ways, it reminded the reporter of "an old-fashioned camp meeting."

Attendees carried their own plates and mugs to meals, which were served from pails. Some amenities had been added since the first Star Camp at Eerde in 1924: pipes had been laid underground to pump hot water into the showers, and huts had been erected to house a post office, a bookstore, a first-aid station, and an information booth. Everything was laid out on a grid, with brick pathways protecting pedestrians from the mud.

Eugenia had never camped before, and she found the camp's vegetarian food "insipid." Washing her own dishes was a novelty. Still, the scene generally enchanted her. More than seventy years later, she still remembered the piney forest air and the birdsong that awoke her in the morning.

The Star Camp featured lectures, dances, and plays, but life there revolved around the evening talks given by Jiddu Krishnamurti, the beautiful young messiah-in-training. The days began with meditation and a brief Krishnamurti discourse. Afternoons were given up to various talks and to games of volleyball. It was at dusk, though, when the camp really came alive.

On one or two nights, rain kept everyone inside. Every other evening, attendees would gather in a big open-air amphitheater, sitting on felled logs surrounding a fifteen-foot pyre. They'd sing folk songs for an hour or more, until, sometime after sunset, Krishnamurti would appear alongside white-haired Annie Besant, the indomitable woman who was both his patron and his disciple. A violinist from Vienna played a piece to set the mood. Krishnamurti, a thirty-one-year-old with a thin, noble face, doleful long-lashed eyes, and an aquiline nose, usually wore Western clothes when in Europe, but for the camps, he donned traditional Indian dress. He would light the pyre while chanting a hymn to Agni, the god of fire. The air would then fill with the delicious scent of burning pine, and the attendees would listen, enraptured, as Krishnamurti began to talk.

His words had a pleasant vagueness that allowed his listeners to project all manner of profundity onto him. In one of his most quoted talks, given the night of July 27, he said, "You give me phrases and cover my Truth with your words. I do not want you to break with all you believe. I do not want you to deny your temperament. I do not want you to do things that you do not feel to be right. But, are any of you happy? Have you, any of you, tasted eternity? . . . I belong to all people, to all who really love, to all who are suffering. And if you would walk, you must walk with me."

On paper, this might seem empty, but Krishnamurti had a quiet charisma that, coupled with the collective will to believe and the exotic atmospherics, drove many attendees into ecstasy. "Whenever He speaks, it is not as if a separate individual was speaking, but as if someone was giving voice to your own greatest thoughts, your own ennobled feelings," wrote one attendee. "And you know that everyone in that mighty audience feels the same—that He is thinking the thoughts of the world, and expressing the hope of the multitude, and after He has spoken you feel you know everyone intimately, however strange before, that you have met in His heart, have lived in His dreams."

It's easy to see why, as she listened to Krishnamurti, Eugenia believed that his was a voice straight from the India of her imagination. Yet Krishnamurti was less a product of India than of Europe. More specifically, he was a product of Europe's obsession with India, a custom-made messiah raised in Theosophy's most elite circles. To understand how Eugenia became Indra Devi, it's necessary to understand the bridge Theosophy created between Eastern and Western spirituality.

By the time Krishnamurti was born in 1895, Theosophy had become deeply established in India. Madame Blavatsky and Henry Steele Olcott's beginnings on the subcontinent had been inauspicious: the first person they stayed with, Arya Samaj president Hurrychund Chintamon, entertained them lavishly but then billed them for everything, even his welcome telegram. Eventually, though, Blavatsky and Olcott were able to find a foothold in both British colonialist and educated Indian society. The English in India, like those in England, loved séances and other supernatural happenings, and Blavatsky obliged them.

Even those who were convinced she was a charlatan found themselves taken with Blavatsky. Her supporters tended to see her as capable of both silly tricks and real magic. That was part of her brilliance: convincing otherwise sensible people that her frauds were but playful embroidery on her deeper engagement with real mysteries. Once one believes this, supernatural claims become unfalsifiable. Indeed, initiates can congratulate themselves on discerning between petty fakery meant for outsiders and authentic wonders. Many gurus (including, decades later, India's most powerful, Sai Baba) would create a similar dynamic among their followers.

It wasn't, of course, just parlor tricks that attracted the British. "The fundamental appeal of theosophy lay . . . in the response it offered to the various dilemmas that constituted the Victorian crisis of faith," writes philosophy professor Mark Bevir. Theosophy came along at a time of widespread European disenchantment. Charles Darwin published *On the Origin of Species* in 1859, fundamentally challenging the biblical account of creation and showing that human existence could be explained without reference to God. Annie Besant, the crusading journalist, feminist, political agitator, and speaker, traveled tirelessly throughout the 1870s, promoting atheism and becoming, in the process, one of the most notorious women in England. In 1887, Friedrich Nietzsche would write, famously, "The greatest recent event—that 'God is dead'; that the belief in the Christian God has become unbelievable—is already starting to cast its first shadows over Europe."

By now, the phrase "God is dead" has been repeated so often that it has lost its meaning, much less its ability to shock, but in the Victorian era, the end of religious certainty was a jarring, even cataclysmic thing. "In the minds of many Victorians, geological discoveries and evolutionary theory had combined to pitch science against Christianity. Theosophy offered them a religious faith that appeared to embrace these discoveries whilst also sustaining a spiritual interpretation of life," writes Bevir.

Some of the leading British figures in India, including A. P. Sinnett, editor of the *Allahabad Pioneer*, and A. O. Hume, who had retired after an illustrious career in the civil service, became active Theosophists. Theosophy's appeal in India, though, was hardly limited to Europeans. Blavatsky and Olcott were extremely popular with many Indians because of their respect for Hinduism and Buddhism, faiths that the colonialists tended to treat with contempt. For generations, British-educated Indians had been taught to regard their traditional religions as no more than barbaric superstition. This left many confused and deracinated. They could never really become British, but schooled in European Enlightenment rationalism, they were estranged from the beliefs of their families.

Theosophy offered a way out of this crisis. It made Indians proud to hear Westerners proclaim that their religion was not only equal to Christianity but superior to it. At the same time, Theosophy refracted Hinduism through a liberal Western lens; it emphasized human equality rather than caste divisions and was consonant with scientific rationalism. It offered an intellectual home for Indians trying to reconcile competing cultures. Among the powerful figures who became Theosophists, at least for a time, were Motilal Nehru and, later, his son, Jawaharlal Nehru, the future Indian prime minister.

From its new headquarters in India, Theosophy spread rapidly in Britain and Europe. Its growth was barely hindered by the scandal that forced Blavatsky to leave the subcontinent. In 1882 she and Olcott had settled on an estate in Adyar, just south of Chennai, which continues as the world headquarters of Theosophy today. Blavatsky had hired a down-on-her-luck old friend, Emma Coulomb, as a housekeeper and taken her into her confidence; Coulomb thus knew Blavatsky's tricks. Increasingly resentful of her menial job, she used that knowledge to try to blackmail the Theosophical Society. Eventually, Coulomb revealed all she knew about the sliding panels and hidden entrances Blavatsky used to "materialize" objects, such as letters from her Himalayan Masters.

Soon after, the Society for Psychical Research, a British group devoted to investigating supernatural phenomena, started looking into Theosophy. The SPR was a respected organization—members included Lord Tennyson, W. E. Gladstone, and William James—with a genuinely open-minded approach to spiritual matters. It even shared some members with the Theosophical Society. The report that emerged from its investigation was enormously damning, though it evinced a sort of respect for Blavatsky's audacity: "For our own part, we regard her neither as the mouthpiece of hidden seers, nor as a mere vulgar adventuress; we think that she has achieved a title to permanent remembrance as one of the most accomplished, ingenious, and interesting imposters in history."

Blavatsky's reputation, particularly in India, was deeply damaged. Under pressure from Olcott, in March 1885 she resigned her official role as the Theosophical Society's corresponding secretary and left for Europe.

Her career, though, was far from over. In London, she settled on Landsdowne Road, supported by wealthy British Theosophists. She started a magazine, *Lucifer*, and as she had in New York, she attracted all sorts of fascinating guests to her home, including Oscar Wilde, W. B. Yeats, and a young law student named Mohandas K. Gandhi. Gandhi read Blavatsky's *Key to Theosophy*, which, he later wrote, "stimulated in me the desire to read books on Hinduism, and disabused me of the notion fostered by the missionaries that Hinduism was rife with superstition."

It was during this period that Blavatsky made her most important convert. In the 1880s, Annie Besant, famed through England and much of the world for her rejection of religion, her daring advocacy of birth control, her Irish republicanism, and her passionate socialism, was having a crisis of faith. Despite her flamboyant apostasy, she had always had a spiritual nature—she'd been an intensely religious child and had married a clergyman, though that union ended in disaster. Even as an atheist, she'd devised freethinking hymnals and replicated the rituals of worship for a secular audience. She threw herself into each new cause with the zeal of a salvation-seeking convert. When these movements failed to deliver the universal brotherhood she longed for, she turned, reluctantly but inexorably, to mysticism.

Besant first encountered Blavatsky when she was asked to review Blavatsky's 1888 opus, *The Secret Doctrine: The Synthesis of Science, Religion, and Philosophy*. Unexpectedly, Besant found that the book spoke to her submerged longings, and she asked a mutual acquaintance for an introduction to the notorious occultist. Blavatsky invited Besant to call on her. It was a fairly ordinary chat, but when Besant went to leave, Blavatsky, staring into her guest's eyes, cried, "Oh, my dear Mrs. Besant, if you would only come among us!"

After that, Blavatsky worked hard to lure Besant into her circle. High-level Theosophists received letters from the Masters about the importance of cultivating her. "Mme. Blavatsky, a skilled amateur psychologist, must have guessed that something of this nostalgia for a belief in the other world still hovered in Mrs. Besant's soul," writes one of Besant's biographers. Besant, meanwhile, fought her attraction to Theosophy, knowing what it would do to her friendships and reputation. Still, the pull was strong, and at one point she heard a divine voice asking, "Are you willing to give up everything for the sake of the truth?" She was.

Imagine if Richard Dawkins announced that he had become a Scientologist—that was the kind of shock Besant's conversion occasioned in England. Her close friend George Bernard Shaw learned of it when he spotted the proofs for an article by Besant titled "Sic Itur ad Astra; or Why I Became a Theosophist," in the offices of the *Star*, a London newspaper. "Staggered by this unprepared blow . . . I rushed round to her office in Fleet Street, and there delivered myself of an unbounded denunciation of Theosophy in general, of female inconstancy, and in particular of H. P. Blavatsky, one of whose books . . . had done all the mischief," he wrote.

Shaw's remonstrance did no good; Besant's mind, once made up, could not be changed. Theosophy, naturally, led her to India, and by the end of the 1890s, she was living most of the year in either Adyar or the home she'd built in Benares—now called Varanasi—a holy city on the banks of the Ganges. Once again, she threw herself into social reform, establishing the Central Hindu College in Benares, which was intended to educate a generation of nationalist leaders steeped equally in Hinduism and modern science. She became a major figure in Indian nationalist politics—in 1917 she would even serve a brief term as president of the Indian National Congress, the body that eventually led the drive for Indian independence.

Blavatsky died in 1891, leaving Besant as the premier public face of Theosophy. When Olcott died in 1907, she became the society's president. Soon after, she declared that Jiddu Krishnamurti, a young Brahmin boy whose father worked on the Adyar grounds, was going to save the world.

Krishnamurti was first identified by Charles Leadbeater, a former Anglican priest who had followed Blavatsky to India many years earlier. Besant's loyalty to Leadbeater was perhaps her greatest human weakness. He was a giant, imposing man with the long beard of a biblical messiah, and he cultivated the image of a powerful clairvoyant. A great fabulist, he would hold the members of his Theosophical circle rapt with elaborate narratives purporting to trace their interwoven past lives, an epic supposedly embedded in a higher plane of knowledge that Theosophists called the Akashic Records. He also had an unfortunate passion for adolescent boys.

Rumors about Leadbeater's involvement with boys in his care

stretched back to his Anglican days. As a Theosophist, he was often in the company of young male disciples, taking some of them along with him on his lecture tours. In 1906, two young men, both sons of American Theosophists, accused Leadbeater of encouraging them to masturbate. A typewritten letter, apparently found in the Toronto flat where Leadbeater had stayed with one of them, was produced. It was written in a simple code; when deciphered, one passage read, "Glad sensation is so pleasant. Thousand kisses darling."

When the scandal erupted, Leadbeater resigned from the Theosophical Society. For Besant, this was more than just a personal disappointment; it was a theological crisis. Leadbeater had encouraged and affirmed her own supernatural visions, and now she was faced with the possibility that they were all merely delusions. Meanwhile, Leadbeater argued that he was merely teaching the boys a kind of psycho-sexual hygiene. In a letter addressed to "My dear Annie," he explained that a man in need of sexual release is "constantly oppressed by the matter," but through self-stimulation, he could create a habit of "regular but smaller artificial discharges, with no thoughts at all in between."

Besant's need to believe him seems to have overpowered her, because she both accepted his explanation and, after becoming president of the society, helped to reinstate him. By 1909 he was once again living at Adyar. There, one evening, he went swimming at the estate's small private beach with some of his young male assistants. That's where he first spied Krishnamurti. Exactly what he saw in the fourteen-year-old is unclear—Krishnamurti was a scrawny, sickly boy, with protruding ribs and a vacant stare, considered something of an idiot by his teachers. According to his lifelong friend and biographer, Mary Lutyens, he was dirty, with crooked teeth and a persistent cough. Nevertheless, Leadbeater expressed awe at his glorious aura and was adamant that he would someday be a great spiritual teacher. Perhaps Leadbeater, despite his apparent pederasty, actually had a measure of mystical insight, because Krishnamurti would indeed go on to a remarkable career as a spiritual sage, particularly once he renounced the Theosophical Society.

Soon, Besant persuaded Krishnamurti's father to give him over to her care, and she founded a separate organization, the Order of the Star in the East, devoted to celebrating and learning from him. She and Leadbeater brought Krishnamurti and his younger brother, Nityananda, to Europe, raising them in a hothouse environment that combined English propriety and fevered religious expectation. Brought up simultaneously to be a gentleman and a savior, Krishnamurti studied both Sanskrit and Shakespeare, took riding lessons, played croquet, and went to the theater, while at the same time learning to give speeches to groups of adoring Theosophists, who found depth in even his most trite utterances. By the time he entered his twenties, he was a shy but beautiful young man who wore suits from the best English tailors and holidayed in the luxurious homes of his many admirers. He had an entourage of upper-class English ladies and young unmarried girls who were sometimes half-jokingly called his Gopis, after the maidens devoted to his namesake, the god Krishna. The fact that he didn't become a monster is itself a minor miracle.

Most of what Krishnamurti knew about Hinduism came to him through Theosophy, though that didn't stop Westerners from imagining that he bore some ineffable Oriental essence. In March of 1926, Fritz Kunz, the leader of the American section of the Order of the Star in the East, lectured about Krishnamurti to two thousand people in Chicago's elegant Hotel Sherman. "The Brahmins of India are gentle and loving, like the Christ, and have the most profound sense of God of any people on earth," he explained. "Therefore, it is natural the new religious leader should come from India. America is too skeptical and too much given to murders."

Krishnamurti was particularly popular among young people—he represented a cosmopolitan, pacifist, healthy spirituality, at once anciently rooted and distinctly modern. This was especially true of the people who flocked to the Star Camps, which were in many ways a decorous precursor to the festivals of the 1960s Western counterculture.

Krishnamurti had a powerful effect on Eugenia. The day after she arrived at the Star Camp, she joined the throng in the main tent for morning meditation. She didn't really know how to meditate, or understand quite what meditation was, so she asked some of the adepts around her. None was very helpful.

Still, she closed her eyes and tried to concentrate. Though there were more than a thousand people in the tent, it was silent except for the sound of wind in the trees outside. Krishnamurti appeared and sat on a small platform, then began to sing a Sanskrit mantra. Eugenia felt odd. Her heart beat quickly, and there was a knot in her throat. She started trembling. As she recalled later, the mantra seemed familiar, though she knew she hadn't heard it before. Around her, everyone was calm, but she felt nervous and dizzy. She'd often been plagued by anxiety attacks, but this was different, stranger. It was, she writes, a kind of "inner shock."

When she opened her eyes, people were moving around her, and she realized that the meditation was over. She stood up and started running until she was in the forest, where she stayed for a while, sobbing, feeling as if all her sadness and fear was pouring out. When she stopped crying, she felt suddenly inexplicably happy, peaceful, and liberated.

That week at the Star Camp was, she writes, "a turning point in my life. Without realizing it then, I had made the first step on the path towards Yoga, with Krishnamurti as my teacher and guide."

Returning to Riga, Eugenia felt completely transformed, with a new sense of tranquility and security. Shortly after she'd come home, she went to dinner at a friend's house. Her friend served her beef, which she'd craved during her meatless days in Ommen. Instead of a nice meal, she saw a slab of dead flesh on her plate, and it disgusted her. She was, she believed, a changed woman.

If Eugenia was different, life in Riga proceeded in much the same way. She kept working in the theater, and Bolm, her fiancé, kept making plans for their future together. More than ever, though, Eugenia felt compelled toward India—and soon a woman came to town who could help her get there.

Alice Adair was a feminist and Theosophist, "an Englishwoman of great dignity, aristocratic bearing, fine taste and cosmopolitan outlook," in the words of a friend. After several years in Australia, she was living at the Theosophical Society's Adyar headquarters. A passionate aesthete, she was an important international champion of Indian art. In 1927 she went to Europe to give lectures on the subject and to present a traveling exhibition of Indian painting, and when she got to Riga, she met Eugenia.

After her European tour, Adair was returning to India in time for a Theosophical convention in December. She seems to have taken Eugenia under her wing and encouraged her to make the trip. With Adair as her guide, Eugenia felt that her dream of getting to India was starting to seem feasible. Only one obstacle remained, though it was a big one: money.

Bolm was impatient with his fiancée's obsession, but he also realized that it was consuming her. He started to think that maybe if she went, she would get it out of her system. Surely India's squalor, crowds, and sickness would disabuse Eugenia of her fantasies. "It's better that she goes," he told her mother, who was even more opposed to the idea. "It could be that this trip will help to destroy all her illusions about India." He bought her a ticket, sending her away for several months with the understanding that they would get married upon her return.

So, on November 17, 1927, Eugenia, traveling alone, boarded a steamship in Naples that was bound for Australia via Ceylon (today's Sri Lanka). As they approached Colombo, Ceylon's capital, after almost a month at sea, "I was in a state of almost delirious ecstasy," she writes. "How many times I had made this journey, travelling in my imagination." In Colombo, she connected with a group of India-bound Australian Theosophists, and before the year's end, she arrived in the port at Madras, now Chennai, in India's southeast. She was finally in the land of her dreams.

If Bolm had seen her arrival, his heart would have sunk. Many Westerners who travel to India are overwhelmed when they get there. The heat is often viscous, like something you swim rather than walk through. Dust assaults you everywhere. The human panoply can be thrilling; there are so many people with unfamiliar faces in unfamiliar clothes: dark and fine-boned southerners, green-eyed Kashmiris, people from the Himalayas who look almost Chinese. Women shimmer in parrot-bright silk saris or light cotton salwar kameezes, jewels sparkling in their noses. There are men in crisp white tunics, men in sarongs, men with wild hair in the shabby loincloths of wandering mystics. Turbans, sometimes brilliantly colored, sit on the heads of bearded Sikhs and mustachioed Rajputs. In the air, there's a constant buzz of mutually unintelligible languages.

The crush of people can be exhilarating, but it can also be terrifying. The poverty is as degraded as anything on earth, the maimed and leprous beggars a reproachful contrast to the opulence of Mughal and Raj architecture. Bands of potbellied urchins, hair turned rust-colored from malnutrition, swarm Westerners. Terrible tropical illnesses thrive in the swampy heat, and in the 1920s, with antibiotics not yet on the market, visiting Europeans often fell seriously ill.

Perhaps Bolm thought that, faced with all this, Eugenia would be cured of her obsession. Instead, she saw only India's enchantments. She was, she writes, "[h]appy beyond measure to be there." Europe would never feel like home again.

PART II

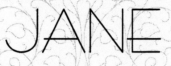
JANE

N 1882, when Colonel Olcott bought the Theosophical Society's property in Adyar, India, for six hundred pounds, it comprised twenty-seven acres, with a single large house flanked by two pavilions. By 1927, when Eugenia arrived toward the end of the rainy season, Theosophy's mecca was a verdant estate of more than two hundred fifty acres, an earnest panreligious fantasia overlaid with Raj gentility. Located seven miles from the South Indian city of Madras on the southern bank of the Adyar River, it was lush with canna lilies, hibiscus, bougainvillea, and oleander, with various groves and gardens named for Theosophical luminaries. Talks and gatherings often took place in a sprawling banyan grove so big it provided shade for thousands. C. W. Leadbeater would stand beneath a canopy of leaves, looking, in the words of one visitor, "like an ancient Druid priest," and lecture about the place of occultism in the new civilization that everyone believed was imminent.

Visitors entered through a carved stone trilithon that Olcott had brought from the ruins of a South Indian temple. On the grounds, there was a Masonic temple and a building for the Liberal Catholic Church, an odd sect (wholly separate from the Roman Catholic Church) that attempted to merge Theosophical ideas with Catholicism's costumes, pomp, and pageantry. A square, columned Parsi temple was under construction, and foundations had been laid for a synagogue and a mosque. Inside the main meeting hall, a cool, whitewashed respite from the pulsating heat outside, the words "There Is No Religion Higher Than Truth" were embossed in gold. Bas-relief figures of Jesus, Buddha, Krishna, and Zarathustra lined the walls, along with an Islamic inscription. There were also smaller images of the Sikh guru Nanak, and of Lao Tse, Confucius, Osiris, Quetzalcoatl, Moses, and others. In a recess behind the speaker's platform stood statues of Olcott and Blavatsky, his hand upon her shoulder. Offerings of flowers were placed before it daily.

During the British Raj, as British rule of the subcontinent was known, employees of the colonial administration generally disdained Indians. Generations of English memsahibs warned new arrivals, "Never shake hands with an Indian, my dear, because you never know where his hand has been." (As historian Margaret MacMillan points out, even after decades of British life in the subcontinent, these English ladies never bothered to learn that Indians generally wash themselves with their left hand and use their right for most everything else.)

Adyar, though, was a different world. There, Indians, Europeans, and Americans all intermingled. One Australian notable, Major General Kenneth Mackay, writes that at Adyar he felt like a citizen of the world, "untrammeled alike by Western or Eastern ecclesiastic or secular tradition."

An unmistakable feminist current ran through Theosophical life. Throughout India, a great many women still remained in purdah, sealed off from the world outside their family homes. To justify their own presence on the subcontinent, British colonialists would sometimes dwell on the lamentable position of India's women, though such Westerners were hardly champions of equality. It had been less than a decade since women in England (or the United States) won the right to vote. In almost all British churches, female ordination was still scarcely imaginable. Adyar, though, was the seat of a spiritual movement founded by one powerful woman and led by another. "Here," writes Mackay, "it has been my privilege to meet women, some of whom have fought and are still fighting a noble battle for the general uplift and liberation of Indian womanhood, struggling not only against age-old religious prejudices but also against official inertia often amounting to passive obstruction."

How could Eugenia help being elated? She'd arrived there alone, directly upon landing in India, but her connection to Adair ensured her embrace. High-level Theosophists were allowed to build their own homes on the Adyar grounds, and Alice Adair's was like a little museum, full of artistic treasures collected on her world travels. There, said a contemporary, "artists and art students met for free exchange of thoughts and ideas."

At the time, Adyar was buzzing in preparation for the annual Theosophical convention, which began in late December and drew more than two thousand people. During the gathering, writes one resident, "Adyar becomes a miniature world, and life becomes thrilling and fascinating . . . Soon the hooting of the horns of taxis and buses, the rattling noise of the jutkas, the tramp of the pedestrians and the shouts of the cartmen, announce the arrival of pilgrims from distant parts of the world—young and old, men and women of all types and classes, in pairs, in groups and in bus-loads."

The sleepy colony was momentarily transformed into a little city, "with bazaars and restaurants, shops and saloons and people of varying castes, colours and creeds." Everywhere, international comrades (misfits, perhaps, in their own societies) reunited happily.

Eugenia had no way of knowing the turmoil that was going on behind the scenes among the Theosophical leadership. In 1927, Krishnamurti was coming into his own as a spiritual teacher, but he was also developing real doubts about Theosophy. In 1925 his brother, best friend, and closest confidant, Nityananda, had died after a long illness. Nitya's death shattered Krishnamurti and accentuated his skepticism about the reality of Theosophy's pantheon of ascended Masters. Theosophical leaders had promised Krishnamurti that the Masters would protect Nitya. When their predictions failed, his mistrust grew.

With the original Theosophical leadership dead, and old age

finally catching up to Annie Besant, the movement was riven by power struggles. Among the new generation of leaders, an atmosphere of febrile and sometimes farcical innovation prevailed, with new rituals, rites, orders, and revelations proliferating like mad. George Arundale, a powerful Theosophist and bishop of the Theosophically inclined Liberal Catholic Church, claimed dramatic communications from the Masters. Many of these messages purportedly announced great leaps in Arundale's own occult status, along with that of his beautiful Indian wife, Rukmini Devi, whom he had married several years earlier, when she was a teenager. Besant was convinced that the revelations were real, and soon announced the coming of the "World Mother," a role meant for Rukmini.

The attempt to create an organization around Rukmini like the one around Krishnamurti elicited widespread ridicule—newspapers predicted the coming of a World Father, a World Infant, and a World Great Aunt—and was soon abandoned. Meanwhile, as the Theosophical Society became increasingly ceremonial and hierarchal, Krishnamurti was developing his own ultra-spare, individualistic approach to spiritual life, which emphasized the need for everyone to find his or her own path, unencumbered by rules and dogmas. Arundale, seeing Krishnamurti as a threat, plotted against him, even at one point trying to convince Besant that dark forces possessed her beloved messiah.

It would be more than a year before any of this burst into the open. Still, at Adyar, some were frustrated by Krishnamurti's vagueness, his refusal to offer definitive answers to their plaintive questions. "Out of those who come to listen, many are up against life's riddles as met within individual or national relations, and seek a new remedy," writes one attendee. "Others come to him as to a dentist for a painless extraction of beliefs he condemns. Some perhaps expect a miracle and have no objection to pick up a ready-made liberation." Krishnamurti refused to give them what they wanted, leaving many restless and unsatisfied.

Not Eugenia, though. To her, everything seemed magical, and her faith in Krishnamurti was absolute. When the annual convention at Adyar was over, Krishnamurti set out on a punishing lecture tour throughout India, and Eugenia joined his entourage. With him, she felt healed. Often when they were to meet, she would compile a list of problems she wanted to speak to him about, only to forget all about them as soon as they were together. "At Krishnamurti's side, everything became clear and perfectly comprehensible," she writes.

Eugenia had an almost supernatural ability to ingratiate herself with people, to make others want to do her favors. Though her family had lost all their belongings, she'd retained her aristocratic manners—indeed, social capital was the only kind she had, and she developed it to the utmost. Her ease among rich and powerful people, her subtle sense of entitlement, made her seem to them like one of their own, and wherever she went they tended to treat her with lavish hospitality. Soon, through Krishnamurti and Adair, she was meeting some of the most fascinating people in India.

With Adair, Eugenia traveled to Calcutta, the onetime British capital. There, they attended an exhibition of young Hindu painters, one of whom was the nephew of the legendary Bengali writer Rabindranath Tagore. Tagore's nephew offered to introduce Eugenia to his uncle. She'd adored Tagore's poems since she was a young girl and was thrilled when she met him at his ancestral home in Calcutta, a house that had long been a center of the city's cultural life.

Thin and aristocratic, with the long, snowy beard of a prophet, Tagore was a giant of Indian nationalism—he wrote India's national anthem, "Jana Gana Mana"—who, like Gandhi, believed that India's strength lay in its rich and ancient spirituality. Yet he was also a world-traveling cosmopolitan, and there was much in the West that he admired. Gandhi's idea of noncooperation with the British pained Tagore; he believed in appropriating the world's riches wherever he found them and in making the best in Indian culture a gift to all humankind.

"All humanity's greatest is mine," he writes. "The *infinite personality of man* (as the *Upanishads* say) can only come from the magnificent harmony of all human races. My prayer is that India may represent the co-operation of all the peoples of the world." At Shantiniketan, a family-owned tract of land about one hundred miles northwest of Calcutta, he created first a school and then a world-class university, Visva-Bharati, which put these ideals into practice. It was deeply and authentically Indian, but also drew from the treasury of worldwide learning. Its Sanskrit motto is "Yatra visvam bhavati ekanidam," which means, "Where the whole world meets in a single nest." Tagore invited Eugenia to visit the school, and she went the next day.

Visva-Bharati was built around three departments: fine arts, music, and Indology, which focused on ancient Indian languages and religious texts. Classes were coeducational and often held in the open air; each teacher had a special tree he lectured beneath. There was an air of cooperation, a blurring of the lines separating teachers and students. "You will find a famous European Scholar studying Bengali from a mere boy," wrote one enthralled visitor. "[Y]ou will also be surprised to find the best minds of India keenly taking language-lessons from visitors from Europe, or following the lectures of young European students on themes like that of the new organized 'Youth movement.'" In the evening, students and teachers would gather to chant Vedic hymns and sit in silent meditation. Nearby, the affiliated Institute of Rural Reconstruction conducted experiments in modern farming methods, intended for the uplift of Indian villagers.

Eugenia adored it. Here was everything she valued—art, spirituality, internationalism, social progress—all in one harmonious place.

She also visited Gandhi's legendary Sabarmati Ashram, outside the city of Ahmedabad, on the western side of the country. Sabarmati, a radically austere attempt at a self-sufficient utopia, was a collection of whitewashed huts surrounded by a few dozen acres of farmland on the banks of the Sabarmati River. There, almost two hundred devotees tried to live according to Gandhi's ascetic ideals. Days began at 4:15 a.m. with prayer, and were later occupied with spinning, weaving, and farming. Everyone, including Gandhi, the most famous man in India, took turns cleaning the latrines. Celibacy was required, even for married couples. Food was strictly bland

and vegetarian; spices or condiments were taboo. Even close friendships were frowned upon, since personal alliances could stand in the way of universal love.

It sounds severe, even cruel, but there could be bliss in it, too. Madeleine Slade, a British admiral's daughter who, like Eugenia, had gone alone to India on a spiritual quest, found rapture in renunciation. Gandhi christened her Mirabehn, or "Sister Mira," and she, like other ashramites, called him Bapu, or "Father." "By God's infinite blessing I had arrived, not at the outer edge of Bapu's activities, but right in the intimate heart of his daily life," Slade writes. "The impact on my emotions was tremendous. From early morning to the last thing at night I lived for the moments when I could set eyes on Bapu."

Though awed by Gandhi, Eugenia lacked Slade's taste for submission and martyrdom, and life at Sabarmati wouldn't have tempted her. (It is unlikely that, in the whole of her almost 103 years, she ever cleaned a toilet.) Yet in visiting Adyar, Shantiniketan, and Sabarmati, she encountered a world in which everyone seemed to be engaged in fantastically earnest, radical experiments in living, in which spirituality and idealism infused daily existence in a way she'd never encountered in Europe. In India, life seemed heightened and profound and full of astonishing possibilities.

As Eugenia crisscrossed India's enormity, it wasn't just rarified company that delighted her. Like many visitors, she was moved by the generosity of ordinary Indians, who invited her into their homes and shared their modest food with her. She discovered that she loved wearing a sari, loved sitting on the ground and using her right hand to eat from banana leaves in the south and metal *talis* in the north, loved the strange spicy dishes that most foreigners avoided. She adored the hot, mazelike bazaars where one could buy spices, scented oils, brilliant silks, armfuls of silver bangles, and a thousand other treasures. And she was taken by the insistent, all-pervading faith of India, the constant sense of transcendence.

Though there were all sorts of regional distinctions, everywhere Eugenia went she was surrounded by images of the divine: sweet, elephant-headed Ganesh; beautiful, romantic Krishna; terrifying Kali with her lolling tongue and garland of human skulls; sacred cows with painted horns wandering in the streets, holding up traffic. Then there were the great serene mosques, with their graceful arches and cool marble; the Buddhist stupas and domed Sikh *gurdwaras*. It all left Eugenia ecstatic, ready to dedicate her life to the country that felt like her spiritual home. " "I wanted to do something for India, live for India, work for India, die for India," she writes.

When, after four months, it was time to go home, despair gripped her. Life in Europe seemed gray and meaningless, but she didn't yet see a way to make India her home. On February 29, 1928, she boarded a slow ship in Bombay for Genoa. Krishnamurti was on the same boat, en route to London, and held discussions with his fellow passengers, but his presence only reminded her of the happiness that was slipping away from her. She lost her appetite and rarely spoke.

From Italy, she took a train to Vienna, where Bolm was waiting for her. He assumed that she'd gotten India out of her system. He was, of course, entirely wrong.

They returned to Riga, and Eugenia began to act again, but she was listless and despondent. As the months passed, her impending marriage loomed like a terrible trap. All she thought about was returning to India, but this appeared impossible. It was one thing, she knew, to go there as a tourist. It was quite another to go there to live, with no independent means or way to support herself. She tried to put the idea aside, but it wouldn't leave her alone. Finally, she grew so desperate that a wild leap into a completely uncertain future began to seem easier than enduring her intolerable present.

She ended her engagement to Bolm, telling him that she no longer loved him and that she planned to return to India for good. He was shocked, and argued with her, but she was firm.

In the spring of 1929, Eugenia turned thirty—which made her, by the standards of the time, a pitiable spinster. But she was relieved to have escaped, at least momentarily, the comfortable prison of matrimony. Part of her craved stability, but it couldn't compete with her need for adventure or her fear, after so many dislocations, of putting down roots anywhere. That summer, she returned to Ommen for the annual Star Camp. It began on August 2, with more than three thousand attendees. Theosophy was, at that point, the most constant thing in Eugenia's life. But on the morning of August 3, Krishnamurti turned his followers' lives upside down.

Krishnamurti had never known anything but Theosophy. It had given him a life of comfort, stimulation, and worldwide adulation. Yet he could no longer pretend to believe in the ascended Masters, in magic, or in the ever-multiplying occult rituals that had come to dominate the Theosophical Society. So, in a speech delivered in the Ommen forest and broadcast on the radio, he renounced the entire mystical edifice that the Theosophists had built around him.

"I maintain that Truth is a pathless land, and you cannot approach it by any path whatsoever, by any religion, by any sect," he proclaimed. No organization should be formed "to lead or coerce people along any particular path." Organizations, he said, are the enemies of truth, slating people into niches, crippling individualism. So, he announced, he was dissolving the Order of the Star in the East.

"For eighteen years you have been preparing for this event, for the Coming of the World Teacher," he said. "For eighteen years you have organized, you have looked for someone . . . who would transform your whole life . . . who would set you free—and now look what is happening! . . . In what manner has such a belief swept away all unessential things of life?"

The Star Order, he argued, was nothing but a crutch, an impediment to true liberation. "[Y]ou have the idea that only certain people hold the key to the Kingdom of Happiness," he said. "No one holds it. No one has the authority to hold that key. That key is your own self, and in the development and the purification and in the incorruptibility of that self alone is the Kingdom of Eternity." He was adamant that he wanted no followers. "You can form other organizations and expect someone else," he said. "With that I am not concerned, nor with creating new cages, new decorations for those cages. My only concern is to set men absolutely, unconditionally free."

The crowd was stunned. "Thousands felt betrayed and insulted," writes Roland Vernon, one of Krishnamurti's biographers. "He had abandoned his post, they thought, and in doing so had capitalised on their misfortune by exposing them as spiritual snobs and pious hypocrites." Annie Besant, who, at eighty-one, had become a bit senile, seemed to be in denial about the fact that her beloved boy was giving up the role she'd created for him. "My fundamental belief in Krishnamurti as the World Teacher makes me more inclined to observe and study than to pronounce an opinion on the method chosen by one whom I consider my superior," she told the Associated Press.

Eugenia's response was contradictory. She admired Krishnamurti's courage and uncompromising individualism, and his denunciation of organizations surely influenced her own lifelong ambivalence about them. Perhaps his willingness to break with the past so decisively bolstered her decision to do the same. Like him, she would become adept at reinvention. At the same time, for the rest of her life, Eugenia never stopped looking for a new messiah.

Her immediate plans, though, remained unchanged. After Ommen, he returned to the Riga apartment she shared with her mother and began to prepare for India in earnest. She sold what was left of her furs, and some jewelry. She said good-bye to her mother, who would soon be moving to Prague for an acting job. Finally, in November, she sailed once again for India via Ceylon, with enough money to last her several months and no real idea what she was going to do.

Despite everything that had happened, Krishnamurti had returned to India with Annie Besant in October 1929 for that year's Theosophical convention. Besant was still like a mother to him—he referred to her as Amma—and he wouldn't officially quit the Theosophical Society until the next year. Eugenia, not knowing quite what to do with herself, decided to go to Adyar as well. The atmosphere there must have been terrifically tense. Most of the Theosophical leadership was nice enough to Krishnamurti in person, but they attacked him behind his back. Ordinary Theosophists bombarded him with pleading questions. Besant, for her part, refused to recognize that things had changed; in a letter to a friend, Krishnamurti complained, "Amma says to me & at meetings, that I am the World Teacher & says she will go on with ceremonies etc. etc.!!" He must, he writes, "get out of all this rot."

Eugenia kept one foot in each camp, continuing to venerate Krishnamurti even as she stayed close to the Theosophical Society. After the end of the convention in Adyar, she installed herself in the cool, park-filled southern Indian city of Bangalore, a couple hundred miles away. There was an active Theosophical scene there, and Eugenia—who had started going by the Anglicized name Jane Peterson, perhaps to fit in better with the Brits who dominated expat society—quickly became a part of it. Most nights, young Bangalore Theosophists would gather to talk, listen to music, and improvise concerts. Eugenia had brought with her from Europe one of the fur-trimmed Russian folk costumes that she used to wear during cabaret performances, and one evening she put it on and danced for her friends. At the time, India had only a few theaters and cinemas, and amateur theatricals were a big part of European social life. She was, it seems, a big hit.

In February, Krishnamurti sailed for California, which would be his base for the rest of his life. Eugenia went to Bombay to see him off and decided to stay for a while. Her fame as a dancer had preceded her, and the Bombay Theosophists arranged for her to give a recital. In the audience was the Indian film director Bhagwati Prasad Mishra, and he was looking for stars.

Nineteen thirty was the peak year for India's silent cinema, which had grown rapidly throughout the 1920s. Indian audiences flocked to mythological stories and adventure fantasias, to social dramas, and even to documentaries about the freedom struggle. Every good-size city had at least one cinema hall, usually with a special *zenana* section, for women in purdah. Traveling cinemas brought movies to smaller towns and village fairs. There would be subtitles in four languages—English, Hindi, Urdu, and a regional language such as Gujarati or Marathi. Often someone would read them out loud for those who were illiterate. Musicians accompanied screenings with harmonium, tabla, and sarangi (or violin). Western movies came to India as well, but Indians much preferred local productions. By the mid-1920s, the beginning of India's intense, vibrant culture of film fandom was in place, and movie stars were the subject of gossip and fascination.

They were not, however, given much respect. The situation was similar to the one Eugenia's mother had once faced: acting was viewed as a thoroughly disreputable profession, and certainly no place for a decent Indian lady. One Hindi magazine ran an article with the headline "Film Actors Are All Pimps and Film Actresses Are All Prostitutes." A piece in *Cinema* magazine lamented, "It is really a perplexing problem as to why those who entertain us every evening through the medium of the silver screen should be denied social standing."

To find actresses, then, directors had to turn either to lower-class dancing girls or to Europeans, Eurasians, and India's Western-orientated Jews. The most famous of all was Ruby Myers, who went by the name Sulochana and often played sexy, surprisingly modern working girls. A daughter of the Baghdadi Jewish community that migrated to India in the 1800s, she'd been discovered while working as a telephone operator. After the smashing success of her 1925 debut, she acted in five or six films a year and earned more than the British governor of Bombay. Other starlets included Renee Smith, a.k.a. Seeta Devi; Iris Gasper, who went by Sabita Devi; and Patience Cooper. In photos, they look like Indian flappers, with their bobbed hair and bindis, their plucked eyebrows and ornate silver jewelry. Sometimes they're pictured wearing saris; other times, they don trousers or calf-baring skirts. Like pre-Code American films, India's silent cinema was racier than what came later; on-screen kissing wasn't banned until the 1940s.

To film director Mishra, a free-spirited young European woman with theatrical training would have been quite a find. So he offered Eugenia the lead role in his new film, *The Arabian Knight*, opposite the dashing young Prithviraj Kapoor, a smoldering Pathan from Peshawar who had come to Bombay two years earlier determined, despite the fury of his policeman father, to make it as a performer. Arriving at Bombay's Gateway of India in 1928 after a two-day, third-class train trip from home, he'd looked up at the sky and pledged, "God, I have come here to become an actor. If you don't make me one here, I will cross the seven seas and go to Hollywood."

He wouldn't have to. In 1929, while working as an extra in the film *Challenge*, Kapoor was spotted by the Jewish starlet Ermeline, who was known as India's Clara Bow. Entranced by the tall, fair, beautiful man with the heroic physique and crackling charisma, she chose him to star opposite her in her next film, *Cinema Girl*, which Mishra directed. Kapoor would go on to become a Bollywood legend, the patriarch of Indian cinema's most famous family. As his biographer put it, "The Nehru-Gandhis and the Kapoors are two dynasties that rule the nation's popular imagination."

At first, Eugenia was skeptical about playing Kapoor's love interest. The female protagonist was supposed to be the most stunning young woman in Baghdad. Eugenia dressed very well and knew how to carry herself, and she'd always had admirers, but she also knew she wasn't a great beauty, and she was almost seven years Kapoor's senior. She told Mishra she didn't think she could pull off the role. Still, he insisted, and she was willing to be convinced. After all, a resumption of her acting career would have seemed a solution to her most immediate problem: how to survive, alone, in India. The money she'd made selling off her valuables in Riga would have been close to running out, and acting was the only job she'd ever done.

Most European women acting in Indian films took Indian names. Mishra suggested Indira Devi—Indira after the daughter of Jawaharlal Nehru, one of the most popular men in India, and Devi because it is the Sanskrit word for "goddess." She agreed. She was only one letter away from becoming Indra Devi; it would take more than another decade to get there.

· CHAPTER 6 ·

I N 1949, the writer, art critic, and longtime Theosophist G. Venkatachalam published a book in Bombay titled, simply, *Profiles*.
It contains sketches, some brief, others several pages long, of the
many extraordinary people he met over the years in India. Among
them are Gandhi, Nehru, Krishnamurti, and Annie Besant. On the
second-to-last page is a paragraph about one "Jean Petersen," a slight
misspelling of Eugenia's Anglicized name. "Jean is an artist of a sort
and thought she could better express herself through dancing as she
knew a little of the ballet before she came here," he writes. "She tried
her hand at many things including starring in Indian films. She hob-
nobbed with Maharajas for a while, and met the Czechoslovakian
Strakaty and married him." Life, writes Venkatachalam, "was one
big adventure for her."

As Venkatachalam's words suggest, as the 1930s progressed, Eugenia was a bit of a dilettante. Because of her charm and her aristocratic bearing, she moved easily through fashionable Indian society.
Thanks to hosts who were happy to have a scintillating woman
around to enliven their gatherings, she often enjoyed a level of opulence that belied her precarious finances. Though she'd come to
India to find transcendence, her energy increasingly went into her
fizzy social life, until finally she found herself in precisely the role

she'd traveled to India to escape. She became defined, first and foremost, as somebody's wife.

Eugenia's Indian cinema career did not last long. Silent films were churned out quickly—few took more than a month—and production on *The Arabian Knight* was short, pleasant, and uneventful. No copy survives—very few silent Hindi films have been preserved—but there are photos. One shows Prithviraj Kapoor in an Arab headdress dipping his costar back and looking into Eugenia's eyes as if about to swoop in for a passionate kiss. She's wearing a gypsy skirt and a long, dark, braided wig. In another photo, she wears a jeweled turban and gazes off into the distance while Kapoor, holding her hand to his heart, stares at her adoringly.

According to Devi's memoirs, when the film came out in 1930, a critic declared her the new star of Indian cinema. Perhaps she could have made more films, but the silent era was coming to an end, and the careers of actresses who weren't fluent in Indian languages would soon wane. Besides, for all but the biggest names, film stardom wasn't hugely lucrative. During the filming of *The Arabian Knight*, Eugenia visited Kapoor at home. He lived with his wife and children in central Bombay, in a nearly bare eight-by-twelve-foot room. His salary was just enough to support his family.

This might be why, shortly after her film's premiere, Eugenia consented to let a friend set her up with Jan Strakaty, the Czech commercial attaché in Bombay. Strakaty, forty-three, was as polyglot as Eugenia—in addition to Czech, he spoke Italian, German, English, French, and some Arabic he'd picked up during four years in Cairo, where he managed a bank branch. His work revolved around business and economics—consulate records describe him as an "excellent force" in opening India to Czech exports. He had little interest in metaphysics and was disdainful of yoga, but according to Eugenia, he was also broad-minded and unconventional, a supporter of women's rights who also sympathized with Hindu nationalism. When he asked Eugenia out to the movies, she tested him by choosing an Indian film, thinking that, like most diplomats she knew, he'd refuse to see it. Instead, he went along happily.

From the start, Eugenia sensed a mutual understanding between them. She believed that they could be close without impinging on each other's autonomy. They could be useful to each other—he needed a charming companion for the never-ending round of diplomatic parties; she needed financial security and a place in a society with little role for single women. So when, shortly after they met, he asked her to marry him, she said yes.

The wedding, as Devi recounted decades later, was a comedy of errors. An enormous storm was tearing through Bombay as they headed toward the civil registry for the low-key ceremony. The howling rain echoed through the magistrate's office, muffling his words. Strakaty was partly deaf thanks to an injury he'd sustained as a soldier during World War I, and kept mishearing.

"Are you ready to marry Miss Jane Peterson?" the judge asked him.

Strakaty thought the judge was asking him if he wanted the ceremony to be held in an Indian language. "Is there any alternative?" he replied. The little wedding party exploded in laughter. Eugenia struggled to stifle her own giggles.

"Do you promise to ensure the interests of your future spouse, as is stipulated in the civil marriage laws?" the judge continued.

"I believe that will be very difficult," Eugenia's fiancé answered, thinking he'd been asked to produce some Czech documents.

At this, Eugenia laughed so hard she started shaking. Thinking she was upset, an alarmed Strakaty turned to her and said, "Don't cry, don't cry, my love!"

In the end, the judge decided to credit the delighted look on Strakaty's face over his words, and he pronounced the two man and wife. They left immediately for a honeymoon in Europe, and as Devi later wrote in her memoirs, "in that manner I began my life as a spouse and ended my artistic path."

She would not flourish in her new role, though that wasn't immediately obvious. Returning to Bombay, Eugenia moved into Strakaty's attractive diplomatic residence. The two of them got along well, not least because Jo, as Eugenia called her new husband, appreciated her independence. He was happy to pass the time playing chess or listening to classical music while she went out dancing with friends her own age. She kept herself in great shape with daily swimming and horseback riding, and studied classical Indian dance with Enakshi Rama Rau, one of the first educated Indian women to appear in Bollywood movies.

Yet the nights full of official parties and dinners were stultifying. When Eugenia wore saris to diplomatic functions, she was met with sneers and snide comments. Often she'd listen, appalled, as various members of the British Raj declaimed with smug certainty on the impossibility of Indian independence.

Having come all the way to India seeking adventure and liberation, Eugenia suddenly found herself with a life that was mundane, conventional, and empty. British diplomatic society in India was famously staid and platitudinous; driven equally by contempt and terror of India, members of the Raj struggled to maintain an exaggerated version of English propriety. Their lives revolved around dinners, social calls, sports, and the British clubs, where night after night expatriates gathered for desultory rounds of drinking, games, and gossip.

The burden of propriety, not surprisingly, fell particularly hard on women. In the 1920s, a professor's wife, newly arrived in the country, was warned by an older woman, "Don't try and be too clever in India. It doesn't go down." Women tended to dress even more conservatively than they would have at home, refusing on principle to make any concession to the enervating heat. Eugenia stood out in her saris or raffish trousers. People gossiped about her friendships with Indians, particularly the nationalists she'd met through Theosophy. One friend even warned her that the police were keeping an eye on her. She ignored such cautions. Diplomatic society posed the real danger to her; her Indian friends helped to keep her sane.

Eugenia was never particularly political, but she felt strongly about Indian independence. She saw how, for Indians, living under a foreign power involved daily insults, even to the aristocrats and celebrated professionals she moved among. A friend of hers was kicked out of his first-class train compartment when an Englishman decided that riding in the same car with an Indian was beneath him. Alongside such routine humiliations was more profound political repression. Indian nationalist leaders were constantly in and out of prison. Police routinely shot at unarmed protesters or charged at them with bamboo *lathis*.

One of Eugenia's close friends was Sarojini Naidu, a huge-hearted poet, activist, and leading figure in the Congress Party. Naidu, two decades older than Eugenia, shared her disdain for asceticism. In Bombay, she would camp out at the opulent Taj Hotel, a domed palace on the waterfront, beside the Gateway to India. There, she entertained lavishly: "Her rooms at the hotel were always crowded with visitors of all sorts, from the princes to the paupers, and she played the hostess in the most princely way," writes one admirer. She was at once fiercely devoted to Gandhi and insouciant toward him; she called him "our Mickey Mouse" or "our ugly angel."

Eugenia recalled visiting Naidu at the Taj one day in 1930. The floor was a riot of bundles and cheap suitcases, and members of the Indian National Congress bustled in and out. "Akka," said Eugenia, using a South Indian term for older sister, "What is all this baggage?" Naidu responded that she was planning on speaking at a meeting the next day and would surely be arrested, and thus was packing for prison. Sure enough, she was jailed for several months in 1930, and then again in 1932, though she was eventually released due to her failing health.

From time to time, Eugenia would herself go to meetings of the Indian National Congress. When she heard that Jawaharlal Nehru was going to be addressing a mass gathering in Bombay, she had to be there.

Nehru, then in his early forties, was Gandhi's oft-imprisoned protégé. The Cambridge-educated son of Kashmiri Brahmins, he was a gorgeous man—something surely not lost on Eugenia—with chiseled features and melting brown eyes. Unlike Gandhi, he was a secularist and an agnostic; he believed that religion was one of India's chief burdens. As a teenager, Nehru had been a Theosophist, inspired by a tutor who had been hired on the recommendation of Annie Besant, a family friend. Besant herself performed his initiation ceremony, and he attended the Theosophical convention in Benares. As he grew older, though, he became contemptuous of his boyhood mysticism. His faith was socialism and anti-imperialism. He was an unlikely tribune for a land as spirit-soaked as India, but he was an electrifying speaker and a brave and brilliant activist. Crowds adored him.

"The young ones among us swore by the vigor of his intellect, the freshness of his outlook, and the radiance of his youth," one Indian politician recalled. "The older folk nodded to one another, wondering at the wise head he carried on his young shoulders; and admiring women agreed with both."

Eugenia was one of those admiring women. Seeing Nehru speak, she was captivated. Not long after, she had the opportunity to meet him when she was invited for dinner at the home of a mutual friend, Jamnadas Dwarkadas, a wealthy Bombay cotton merchant and prominent Theosophist. At another friend's suggestion, she performed a dance for Nehru, and afterward her hosts seated her beside him, on a low Indian divan. Eugenia plied him with questions about how he had developed the spiritual fortitude to take on the British Empire and to survive his many stays in prison. He told her that, more than anything, what had saved him when he was locked up was yoga.

It turned out that despite his secularism, Nehru had come to swear by hatha yoga's physical and mental benefits. When Eugenia met him, he'd recently been released after his fifth prison term. Incarcerated, he found it a constant struggle to maintain both his health and his spirit. "The object of jail appears to be first to remove such traces of humanity as a man might possess and then to subdue even the animal element in him so that ultimately he might become the perfect vegetable!" he wrote to his sister Nan. "Soil-bound, cut off from the world and its activity, nothing to look forward to, blind obedience the only 'virtue' . . ." Amid the squalor, degradation, and hideous boredom of prison, practicing asana helped him maintain his strength and equilibrium. Every morning, he'd spend five or ten minutes in shirshasana, or headstand, a practice he maintained for much of his life. "It's a complete reversal of the normal situation," he told one journalist. "The body is forced to adapt itself to new conditions."

Later he would write about yoga in *The Discovery of India*, penned during another imprisonment. "The *Yoga* system of Patanjali is essentially a method for the discipline of the body and the mind leading up to psychic and spiritual training," he writes. He praised yoga's experimental, empirical nature—it is, he writes, "a method for finding things out for oneself rather than a preconceived metaphysical theory of reality or of the universe."

Always a rationalist, Nehru was particularly interested in the physical side of yoga, which had only recently emerged from long obscurity and disrepute. Like many of his contemporaries, he saw it in the context of Indian nationalism, as a superior indigenous type of physical culture. "This old and typical Indian method of preserving bodily fitness is rather remarkable when one compares it with the more usual methods involving rushing about, jerks, hops, and jumps which leave one panting, out of breath, and tired out," he writes. Indians engaged in sports and pastimes such as wrestling, swimming, fencing, and riding, but "the old *asana* method is perhaps more typical of India and seems to fit in with the spirit of her philosophy."

Eugenia had told Nehru, a bit flirtatiously, that she wanted a picture of him but didn't like any of those for sale in the markets. The next day, he mailed her a photo of himself that he thought was flattering. (Until the end of her life, she kept a picture of him taken at around this time. In it, he wears a white tunic and a white cap. His hands are clasped behind his back, and there's a hint of a melancholy smile on his lips.) "As you seemed to be interested in my pictures I am taking the liberty of sending you a copy," he wrote. "It was a delight to see you for dinner yesterday. I hope the pleasure will be repeated." He seems to have thought she was single, since the letter is addressed to "Miss Peterson." In subsequent letters, he just called her "Jane."

"Certainly I would like to see you again," he wrote to her a little while later. "Are you free tomorrow? If so come in the morning about 8:30 am. Today I have got a number of meetings and interviews." Soon they developed a warm friendship. She saw him when he passed through Bombay, and she made many trips to Allahabad, the city where he was born and where he continued to be based. There, she stayed at the home of a nearby maharaja and frequented Anand Bhawan, the Nehru family mansion, a luxurious forty-two-room estate that often served as the nerve center of the Indian independence movement. It was so crowded with admirers, it seemed more a place of pilgrimage than a private home.

Once, she arrived when Gandhi was there. It was one of the Mahatma's days of silence, and he was sitting on a carpet under a pergola in Nehru's garden. Nehru took her by the hand and brought her to the Mahatma's side. Sitting by the small, frail-seeming, immensely strong man in the loincloth, looking into the merry eyes behind his round spectacles, "I felt that I was being initiated into a sacramental mystery," she writes.

Being close to such extraordinary people was exhilarating, but it also reminded her how meaningless her own life had become. She'd traveled to India to pursue the secrets of yoga, but had not gotten anywhere close. Instead, she'd ended up a society wife. She had friends who were fully engaged with life's deepest problems, while she watched from the sidelines, feeling irresolute and frivolous. "Was this why I had come to India?" she writes. "To become a popular hostess and party-goer?"

Other women filled their lives with children, but Eugenia had no interest in motherhood, and she considered the fact that she'd never become pregnant to be an enormous blessing. (In her last years, reproductive rights was one of the few political issues she took a strong stand on.) She wanted to devote herself to her own projects, her own quest, but what was that? She no longer knew. She was thirty-two and lost.

Soon she was sick as well. Later, she would describe her illness in occult terms, though a more plausible explanation lies in her terrible ennui. Sometime in 1932, Jo went south on a hunting trip, and

Eugenia was having dinner with a friend. He seemed torpid and unwell. Then, on their way home, he doubled over in pain. Eugenia had read about so-called "Magnetic Healing" in *Fourteen Lessons in Yogi Philosophy and Oriental Occultism*, by Yogi Ramacharaka, a.k.a. William Walker Atkinson. (That she still believed this book was authentic testifies to how little she'd managed to learn about yoga during her first years in India.) The yogic healer, writes Ramacharaka, "passes his hand over the body of the sick person, and by an effort of will, or strong desire, generates within himself a strong supply of Prana which he passes out to the patient."

Eugenia was inspired to try it out. They went to her friend's house, where, just as Ramacharaka instructed, Eugenia had him sit in an armchair while she moved her hands above his body in circles, concentrating as hard as she could on making him better. Then she gave him some magnetized water, a remedy popular in Theosophical and other natural-healing circles.

The next day, as she later told the story, her friend called to say that he felt much better. She, however, awoke with a terrible pain in her chest, one that refused to subside. She saw a doctor, but he could do nothing for her but give her pain pills and prescribe liver injections, which she consented to despite her vegetarianism. She went home, took to her bed, and stayed there day after day, convinced that she'd absorbed her friend's bad energy into herself. When Jo returned, he was horrified to see how ill she was, though he didn't agree with her on the cause. He arranged to take her to Europe to confer with cardiologists on the Continent.

None of them, however, could find anything wrong with her, and after six months, the couple returned to Bombay. As the hot season began its annual siege on the capital, Eugenia deteriorated. From her description of those days, it sounds like she was being crushed by a combination of clinical depression and anxiety attacks, perhaps like those she'd had as a child. She was nervous, irritable, tearful, and listless. She felt too tired to accompany her husband to most of his engagements, or to swim, dance, or ride horseback. She gained weight, and her skin looked dull and lined, though she scarcely had the energy to care. Once so audacious and vibrant, now she alternated between impotent misery and dull resignation.

For the next four years, she moved in and out of this wretched fugue. Occasionally, she would rouse herself to attend a party or take a dance lesson, but most of the time she was too exhausted to do anything at all. She'd become a sickly housewife, her ambitions utterly circumscribed.

This sort of thing, of course, happened to many women— decades later, Betty Friedan would catalyze second-wave feminism by describing the plight of intelligent women who were driven half-crazy by the boredom, banality, and lack of purpose in their lives. For middle-class European women in India, the stifling heat and frequent illnesses compounded the housewife's languor. "Less energetic women lapsed into an almost permanent lethargy," writes historian Margaret MacMillan. Eugenia had always been plenty energetic, but as her life veered into a cul-de-sac, she felt spent.

Given her esoteric interests, it's not surprising that she viewed her troubles in occult terms—and it was through occultism, of a sort, that she eventually found relief.

It came not in India but in Prague, where she'd gone on vacation with her husband. There Strakaty, as the commercial attaché, had to go see a new kind of Czech handloom, presumably for possible export to India. Eugenia accompanied him, and the inventor dragooned her into taking a weaving lesson with him. She wanted to get out of it—she had no interest in handicrafts and couldn't even sew a button—but somehow couldn't extricate herself. During the class, she had some sort of nervous attack. As it turned out, one of her fellow students was studying to be a doctor. Feeling her pulse racing, he had her lie down, gave her some brandy, and put a cold compress on her chest.

Afterward, she told him her whole history, starting with her attempt at healing her friend. The medical student, Mr. Rypka, was interested in yoga—or, at least, what he understood to be yoga—and appalled by the way she'd attempted to dabble in the body's hidden powers without proper training. "Just like electric energy, they can cure or kill—it all depends on the way you use them," he told her. He asked her if she'd consulted a yogi about her illness and was surprised when she said no. Upon thinking about it, she was surprised as well. Why hadn't she? She wasn't sure. Perhaps her depression had eclipsed her initiative.

Rypka resolved to treat her himself—indeed, he promised he could cure her in seven days. She was skeptical but willing. Like her, it seems that he was influenced by Ramacharaka. During five fifteen-minute sessions, he rubbed his hands together to produce heat and electricity and then passed them over her body. After each session, she slept deeply and awoke feeling improved. On the final day, she told him she felt much better, though not completely well. He promised her that by the next day she would.

"The next morning I woke up with a wonderfully light feeling and a sense of well-being," she writes. She felt suffused with health and ran around dancing and singing with relief and joy. Her husband didn't take this revival seriously and expected her to revert, but Eugenia was confident that she'd made a miraculous recovery.

One needn't have faith in the validity of Rypka's methods to believe that he made Eugenia feel much better. Psychosomatic maladies are particularly responsive to faith healing. Rypka gave her confidence in her future by reawakening an old passion, one that she'd given up on ever realizing. Once again, she had a goal in life. Returning to Bombay, Eugenia was determined finally to start studying yoga seriously. Finding the right teacher, though, wouldn't be easy.

N AUGUST OF 1932, more than five hundred wandering Hindu holy men, or sadhus, camped out on Bombay's Chowpatty Beach after attending a festival in the city of Nasik, about one hundred miles away. (In order to get rid of them, Nasik officials had offered free transportation out of town.) As the weeks went by and the ash-smeared mendicants, some entirely naked, showed no sign of leaving, Bombay authorities got worried. They couldn't forcibly remove the sadhus without creating a backlash among poor Indians who admired them, but much of the middle class found them mortifying, while the Europeans were alternately titillated and appalled. At a meeting about the problem, one municipal official fretted that crowds of people were going to see the holy men. "No respectable people will go there," responded another, M. A. Karanjawalla.

Over lunch one day, a German girlfriend of Eugenia's proposed an outing to see the sadhus, and Eugenia immediately agreed. So, on a steamy summer evening, with the lights of Bombay glowing behind them, they joined the carnivalesque throngs wandering "through the rows of mushroom-like umbrellas stuck in the ground," each one sheltering a wild-looking ascetic. They were, as far as Eugenia could tell, the only Europeans there.

Eugenia was fascinated. The men were naked or nearly so, their skin smeared with holy ash. Some were bent into impossible-seeming contortions or frozen in precarious balances. "They resembled a group of jugglers and acrobats in gray tights and make-up," she wrote. "Their fantastic coiffures towered on their heads like huge birds' nests, stiff as wigs and yellowish from the application of cow dung."

One of them stood on his head the entire time they were there.

"Why on earth is he doing that?" Eugenia asked.

"To please God," answered a bystander.

Eugenia made a remark about God's peculiar taste and said she'd always imagined genuine Indian yogis quite differently from these showmen.

"But these are not yogis," exclaimed a passing student. "These filthy loafers and mischief makers only ruin India's good name with foreigners such as yourselves."

Such was the reputation, during her first years in India, of hatha yoga, the body-centric yoga practice Eugenia would later make famous. It was widely seen as the province of magicians, con men, and sideshow contortionists. Even champions of Indian religion typically dismissed it. When educated people, whether Indian or Western, spoke respectfully of yoga, they usually meant a system of breathing, meditation, and philosophy, not physical postures.

Madame Blavatsky had described the "torture and self-maceration" of hatha yoga as "the lower form of Yoga." Swami Vivekananda, the Bengali monk who became an iconic figure of the Hindu renaissance, was largely dismissive of it. Vivekananda's hugely influential 1896 book *Raja Yoga* inspired educated Indians and catalyzed a Western fascination with Indian spirituality that has yet to abate. But *Raja Yoga*—which means "Kingly Yoga"—dismisses hatha yoga. "We have nothing to do with it here, because its practices are very difficult and cannot be learnt in a day, and, after all, do not lead to much spiritual growth," he writes. "Many of these practices—such as placing the body in different postures—you will find in the teaching of Delsarte and others. The object in these is physical, not spiritual." (He is referring to François Delsarte, a French acting teacher who inspired an international vogue for spiritualized gymnastics.)

Yet, as the 1930s progressed, hatha yoga's reputation began to change rapidly. Thanks to a few brilliant innovators, it was being transformed from a lurid, threatening relic into a wholesome indigenous science of health and longevity. And Eugenia, on a quest to free herself from her heart-palpitating nervous attacks, would find herself right at the center of the hatha yoga renaissance.

Yoga as a system of physical fitness is, contrary to conventional wisdom, a fairly modern phenomenon. If few people realize that, it's partly because the word *yoga* is so labile, creating a false sense of continuity among many distinct practices. As the great scholar of religion Mircea Eliade writes, "The word *yoga* serves, in general, to designate any *ascetic technique* and any *method of meditation*." When people say "yoga," they can be talking about many different things.

It is true that Indians have been doing yoga for millennia, but their practices didn't necessarily have anything in common with yoga as currently understood by the West, as a series of poses and breathing exercises designed to strengthen the body and calm the mind. Much like Theosophy, modern yoga is a hybrid of ancient and contemporary ideas, an East-West fusion.

The most well-known text of classical yoga is *The Yoga-Sutra of Patanjali*, which scholars generally date to somewhere between 200 BC and AD 250, though the techniques it presents are thought to be far older. References to the philosopher Patanjali are common in contemporary Western yoga classes, which might give students the idea that their practice is rooted in his writing. It isn't. *The Yoga-Sutra* is a short text, comprising 196 aphorisms. The sum total of its teaching about yoga poses is this, in scholar Georg Feuerstein's translation: "The posture [should be] steady and comfortable. [It is accompanied] by the relaxation of tension and the coinciding with the infinite [consciousness-space]."

Patanjali's yoga is neither an exercise regimen nor a medical modality. It is a practical philosophy—and arguably a quite pessimistic one. Starting from the assumption that human life is full of intolerable suffering and that suffering derives from mental activity, it offers a schema for escaping the pain of worldly existence through the dissolution of the ego and the cessation of thought. As the second stanza of the *Yoga-Sutra* puts it, *Yogas citta vrtti nirodhah*, which Feuerstein translates as "Yoga is the restriction of the fluctuations of consciousness."

In their diagnosis of the human predicament, Patanjali and other classical yoga philosophers had some of the same insights that would later spawn existentialism and psychoanalysis. They understood the way our perceptions shape our reality, and they were profoundly concerned with the anguish of being trapped by one's thoughts. They elaborated practical techniques, particularly breathing and concentration exercises, to aid adepts in observing the workings of their own minds, a sort of self-psychoanalysis or even self-hypnosis.

Mystics from every religious tradition report rapturous experiences of union with the divine and direct perception of numinous truths that transcend language and logic. Yoga elaborates a rational path for inducing such suprarational states. That's why so many who developed a taste for altered states of consciousness in the 1960s found yoga congenial. It can be, as Feuerstein subtitles one of his books, "The Technology of Ecstasy."

It's clear why so many iconoclastic Western thinkers have been electrified by yogic wisdom. "Depend upon it, rude and careless as I am, I would fain practice the yoga faithfully . . . to some extent, and at rare intervals, even I am a yogi," Henry David Thoreau wrote in an 1849 letter. Many psychoanalysts, particularly Carl Jung, saw the parallels between their own disciplines and yoga philosophy; Jung called yoga "one of the greatest things the human mind has ever created."

Nevertheless, classical yoga clashes with the deepest values of modern individualism. The point of Patanjali's philosophy is to reject and transcend this world, not to function more easily within it. His yoga is a tool of self-obliteration more than self-actualization. Feuerstein, a great admirer of Patanjali, is adamant about this. Patanjali's idea of the conquest of the ego "presupposes that we turn our back on all things of the world, on life itself," Feuerstein writes. "Patanjali's is not a way of living *in* the world free from fear of death or loss of any kind, but of acquiring an other-worldly dimension of existence where properly speaking it no longer makes any sense to talk of fear or its removal. The transformation of human nature as envisaged in Classical Yoga is entirely a process of negation of everything that is ordinarily considered as typically human." The archetypical yogi, after all, was a half-naked hermit.

The fact that yoga is now seen as a route toward individual development and a more efficacious life in the world is thus a historical irony. Eugenia would play an important role in this conceptual transformation.

While classical yoga has little to say about asana practice, in medieval times a clear yogic focus on the body, and on techniques for preserving it, emerged. Hatha yoga, as the physical side of yoga is called, was originally the name of a discipline practiced by an order of twelfth-century ascetics known as the Kanphata yogis. As Eliade explains, however, "the term soon came to be the collective designation for the traditional formulas and disciplines that made it possible to attain [the] perfect mastery of the body."

It is in the hatha yoga texts—*The Gheranda Samhita*, *The Hatha Yoga Pradipika*, and *Shiva Samhita*—that asanas first play a major role. The first of these books describes thirty-two poses; the second, fifteen; and the third mentions eighty-four, though only four, the seated poses *Siddhasana*, *Padmasana*, *Paschimottananasana*, and *Sukhasana*, are elaborated upon. Most of the asanas described in these texts are either seated or supine; there's no mention of now-familiar standing sequences such as *surya namaskar*, or sun salutations, in any ancient work.

Hatha yoga combined elements of Patanjali's yoga with tantra, a transgressive, occult tendency within Hinduism that turns upside down traditional concerns with purity. Tantra is itself a complex, multilayered tradition, but Wendy Doniger, one of the leading Western scholars of Hinduism, writes that tantric texts and rituals typically include "worship of the goddess, initiation, group worship, secrecy, and antinomian behavior, particularly sexual rituals and the ingesting of bodily fluids." Inversion and reversal are hugely important within tantra. Substances that classical Hinduism regards as polluting are transubstantiated and become sacred; one variant of tantra prescribes ritual ingestion of the "Five Jewels": semen, urine, feces, menstrual blood, and phlegm.

In hatha yoga, it's the very functions of the body that are inverted. In his eccentric but fascinating study of yoga and Zen, Arthur Koestler points out that in hatha yoga, if "the function of an organ can be reversed, this will be done, whatever the effort." Organs meant for excretion are instead trained to take substances in—*Vajroli Mudra*, described in *The Hatha Yoga Pradipika*, involves sucking released semen, or *bindu*, back into the urethra. ("The Yogi who can protect his *bindu* thus, overcomes death; because death comes by discharging *bindu*, and life is prolonged by its preservation.") Meanwhile, organs meant for intake—the eyes, the mouth, the nose—"must be blocked, locked, sealed to the world. If this cannot be done completely, the functions will at least be partially suspended: breath, heart-pulse, pulse."

Pranayama, the control of the breath, is thus something much more significant than simple deep breathing. *The Hatha Yoga Pradipika* instructs in the practice of *Khechari Mudra*, in which the yogi cuts the tendon connecting the tongue to the bottom of the mouth, then works, over time, to lengthen it. Eventually, the yogi can push the tongue behind the soft palate and use it to direct breath from one nostril to another, or shut the breath off completely. "He who knows the Khechari Mudra, is not troubled by diseases, is not stained with karmas, is not snared by time," *The Hatha Yoga Pradipika* promises.

Hatha yoga's ultimate aim is the raising of sacred kundalini energy. Often envisioned as a snake that lies coiled at the base of the spine, kundalini energy represents man's dormant (and sometimes supernatural) potential. Hatha yoga exercises are meant to awaken it and then force it up a channel that runs along the spine to the crown of the head. As it rises, the energy traverses the body's chakras, or energy centers, activating latent powers as it goes.

There's an element of magic here that gets lost if you interpret the texts as simple guides to better health. Certain asanas are said to confer *siddhis*, or "supernatural powers." The complex mystical physiology elaborated on in yoga texts—the subtle body comprised of chakras and *nadis*, or "channels"—does not necessarily correspond with the empirical, physical body. In other words, it's a mistake to see the chakras merely as analogies to nerve plexuses. "'Subtle physiology' was probably elaborated on the basis of ascetic, ecstatic, and contemplative experiences expressed in the same symbolic language as the traditional cosmology and ritual," writes Eliade. "This does not mean that such experiences were not *real*; they were perfectly real, but not in the sense in which a physical phenomenon is real."

When yoga is seen this way, mixing up mystical physiology and concrete human anatomy would be a category error akin to performing a blood transfusion with wine from the Eucharist. Yet this sort of categorical confusion about the difference between mystical, symbolic language and secular literalism would become hugely important in the development of yoga-as-exercise.

Indian spirituality has long valued feats of asceticism, and asanas were involved in religious austerities as well as alchemical experiments. The seventeenth-century French physician and traveler François Bernier writes of naked, ash-smeared "Jauguis," some dragging heavy chains, others spending hours in handstands and other postures "so difficult and painful that they could not be imitated by our tumblers." The point of these exercises was devotional rapture and the destruction of individual subjectivity more than the enjoyment of robust good health.

That said, there was an important physical fitness element in the lives of many hatha yogis. These men—and they were overwhelmingly men—were often far from the peaceable sages of the Western imagination. In fact, large numbers of them were fighters, akin in some ways to Shaolin monks. As the scholar Mark Singleton writes, from the fifteenth century until the beginning of the nineteenth century, "highly organized bands of militarized yogins controlled trade routes across Northern India." Many formed mercenary militias. According to G. S. Ghurye, a leading Indian scholar, as many as seven thousand naked ascetics used to march, armed with spears, shields, bows, and arrows, at the head of the Jaipur Army.

To prepare their bodies for fighting, these militant yogis adopted punishing exercise regimens that were, as Ghurye puts it, "almost the counterpart of the military drill that a regular regiment receives as a part of its training to keep it in trim." It's possible that some of the exercises now associated with hatha yoga had their origin in this sort of combat training, something separate from the yogis' religious practice. That, writes Singleton, would help "explain the apparent discrepancy between postures described in medieval *hatha* yoga texts and the kind of postural practice ascribed to hatha yoga by modern innovators."

The British Raj was mostly able to pacify India's yogin armies, driving the yogis to society's margins. "No longer able to make a living by trade-soldiering, large numbers were forced into lives of yogic showmanship and mendicancy, becoming objects of scorn for many sections of Hindu society, and of voyeuristic fascination or disgust for European visitors," Singleton writes. They became, in other words, like the yogis Eugenia saw on Chowpatty Beach.

Such yogis were despised by orthodox Hindus and many modern reformers alike. The former reviled their impurity and disregard for caste. The latter saw them as relics of a superstitious, even barbarous, past they were eager to leave behind. Thus even as yoga philosophy enjoyed renewed international respect around the turn of the twentieth century, hatha yoga remained in disrepute—until the global craze for physical culture rehabilitated its reputation.

༄

If Swami Vivekananda wasn't a hatha yogi, he nevertheless helped set the stage for the hatha yoga revival. A crucial bridge between

India and the West, Vivekananda was the first Indian to turn the traditional missionary relationship on its head, bringing a modernized version of Hinduism to America. At the same time, he helped transmit back to India Western ideas about the spiritual value of physical fitness, ideas that would inform the reinvention of hatha yoga.

Vivekananda's arrival in the United States for the World's Parliament of Religions in 1893 was a signal event in the history of American alternative spirituality. The parliament was held in conjunction with the Chicago World's Fair, an unprecedented spectacle erected to celebrate the four-hundredth anniversary of Christopher Columbus's arrival in the Americas. Pavilions—the Electricity Building, the Palace of Mechanic Arts, the Agricultural Building—celebrated the country's innovation and abundance. Frederick Law Olmsted, the landscape designer who created Manhattan's Central Park, turned the grounds into an American Venice, replete with canals, lagoons, and gondolas. The world's first Ferris wheel conducted amazed visitors heavenward. On the Midway, sideshows and cultural curiosities beckoned: fortune-tellers, magicians, and the famous Cairo Street, with its bejeweled camels and scandalous belly dancers.

The World's Parliament of Religions partook of the fair's universalizing spirit, its optimistic American assumption that all the world's faiths could be gathered together, each contributing its own particular treasures. "Religion, like the white light of Heaven, has been broken into many-colored fragments by the prisms of men," wrote the conference chair. "One of the objects of the Parliament of Religions has been to change this many-colored radiance back into the white light of heavenly truth."

Over two weeks in September, the parliament brought together representatives from most of the world's religions—Jews and Christians, Hindus and Muslims, Buddhists, Parsis, Zen masters, Confucianists, and Shintoists. Mary Baker Eddy, the founder of Christian Science, sent a speech to be read in absentia, and thousands packed the hall to hear it. Many attendees were Theosophists; even Mohammed Webb, an American convert who represented Islam, identified with the society. Altogether, one hundred fifty thousand people attended.

The undisputed star of the conference was thirty-year-old Swami Vivekananda. Stout but handsome, with a regal, leonine bearing, he was "clad in gorgeous red apparel, his bronzed face surmounted with a huge turban of yellow," as one attendee described him. With a sharp wit and a delightful Scottish brogue courtesy of the mission school where he'd learned English, he was perfectly attuned to the parliament's universalizing religious spirit.

A devoted Indian nationalist, he'd been sent to the United States to plead for an end to the Christian missionary activity that was subverting his country's religious traditions. (One of his patrons was the Maharaja of Mysore, whose son and successor would later have a major impact on Eugenia's life.) Vivekananda was a devotee of Ramakrishna Paramahamsa, an ecstatic mystic and worshipper of the goddess Kali. He was also dedicated to defending the reputation of Hinduism abroad, and to that end, he reimagined his master's teachings in a way that was very much in line with Western liberal religious sentiments. His hybrid philosophy was deeply influenced by American transcendentalism, which was itself shaped by romantic conceptions of Indian thought, one of those cross-cultural Ouroboroses found throughout the history of yoga in the West.

Vivekananda well understood how India (and he himself) could benefit from the veneration of searching Westerners. As he wrote in a letter to the Maharaja of Mysore, educated Americans had become "disgusted" by theories of "a big tyrant God sitting on a throne in a place called Heaven, and of the eternal hell fires." His version of the Vedanta school of Hindu philosophy, which saw God not as a capricious father but as "our highest and perfect nature," could speak to American intellectuals, filling the void left by religious disenchantment.

Further, he believed, the more that sophisticated Westerners came to admire Indian religion, the more they would support Indian independence. "By preaching the profound secrets of the Vedanta religion in the Western world, we shall attract the sympathy and regard of these mighty nations," Vivekananda wrote to one journalist friend, "maintaining for ever the position of their teacher in spiritual matters, and they will remain our teachers in all material concerns." Elsewhere, he put it a bit more crudely. "As our country is poor in social virtues, so this country is lacking in spirituality," he wrote. "I give them spirituality, and they give me money."

In Chicago, Vivekananda presented Vedanta as essentially an ancient, venerable antecedent to American New Thought, the popular mind-over-matter doctrine. He invited Americans to slough off Judeo-Christian ideas of sin and guilt: "Allow me to call you, brethren, by that sweet name, heirs of immortal bliss—yea, the Hindu refuses to call you sinners . . . Sinners? It is a sin to call a man so; it is a standing libel on human nature."

Americans embraced Vivekananda's vision of salvation through self-realization. The *New York Herald* called him "undoubtedly the greatest figure in the Parliament of Religions." Following the parliament, he signed up with a lecture bureau and spent months traveling around the country for speaking engagements. Disciples began to collect around him; in 1895 he initiated his first two Western sannyasins, or "renunciants." When his book *Raja Yoga* was published in 1896, it sold out in months.

Vivekananda's modernized version of Vedanta would have a huge impact on American New Age religion, particularly in Los Angeles, where the Vedanta Society that his followers opened would attract expat devotees such as Christopher Isherwood and Aldous Huxley. Frank Baum, the Theosophist author of *The Wizard of Oz*, first heard Vivekananda speak in Chicago and was deeply affected by him; Baum's biographer Evan I. Schwartz argues that the quests of Dorothy, the Scarecrow, the Tin Man, and the Cowardly Lion are all allegories for the four yogic paths that Vivekananda elaborated.

Almost as important as the ideas that Vivekananda brought to the United States, though, were the ones he brought home to India.

Vivekananda had come to America at the height of the craze for what was then called physical culture. It started in the mid-1800s, when experts in both Europe and the United States grew worried that sedentary lives born of industrialization were making people weak and neurotic. An evangelistic passion for the wholesome, curative powers of exercise and health food was thus born. The idea of "muscular Christianity" infused the quest for bodily strength with religious valor.

American newspapers and magazines hailed men such as doctor and homeopath Diocletian Lewis, a feminist, temperance activist, and abolitionist who promoted a gymnastic-based "movement cure" for female invalids. John Harvey Kellogg, inventor of corn flakes, ran the famous Battle Creek Sanitarium in Michigan, which treated famous patients such as President William Taft and aviatrix Amelia Earhart with a regime of vegetarian food, breathing exercises, gymnastics, massage, and enemas.

Toward the end of the nineteenth century, the Prussian strongman Eugen Sandow became an international celebrity and sparked the modern bodybuilding movement. While Vivekananda was in Chicago for the World's Parliament of Religions, Florenz Ziegfeld, then an unknown impresario whose father ran a struggling Chicago nightclub, made his name by putting Sandow onstage, to awed reviews: "Sandow looks and feels more like a steel machine than a human being," wrote the *Chicago Tribune*. "[W]hen he holds three horses on his chest, to say nothing of a teeterboard on which the animals stand, people forget to applaud, they hold their breaths and wonder."

Vivekananda was strongly affected by the physical culture movement, even if he didn't do much exercise himself. If Westerners had pioneered muscular Christianity, he sought to create a muscular Hinduism, believing that Indians needed physical strength to gain their independence. After all, British domination was often justified in terms of physical superiority over sickly, effeminate subalterns, and Indians had internalized this hierarchy. One popular children's chant from the Indian state of Gujarat went, "Behold the mighty

Englishman / He rules the Indian small / Because being a meat-eater / He is five cubits tall."

For Vivekananda, as for others who followed him, becoming strong was a crucial step toward becoming free. Indeed, he was even willing to jettison the most profound Hindu taboos in the name of bodybuilding. An unrepentant beef eater, he told one disciple, "The entire country has become crowded with sickly, dyspeptic, vegetarian ascetics . . . Now we have to make our countrymen enterprising by feeding them fish and meat." Vivekananda also made a crucial link between controlling the body and controlling the mind, asking in one dialogue, "How will you struggle with the mind unless the physique be strong?"

Physical culture spread rapidly in turn-of-the-century India, closely linked to Indian nationalism. When the bodybuilder Sandow traveled to India in 1905, as part of a triumphant world tour, he was a sensation. As he stepped off the train at Calcutta's Howrah Station, he found hundreds of people waiting to greet him, and when he appeared in theaters and tents around the country, the standing-room-only crowds were "electrified," in the words of the *Times of India*. Local newspapers heaped praise on him, and one wealthy Parsi businessman offered him ten thousand pounds if he stayed on in the country. The Maharaja of Baroda displayed a life-size plaster cast of Sandow in his personal museum.

Sandow assured his Indian audiences that with proper training, they, too, could become strongmen. "The native Indians have a fine foundation for the building of large, physical men," he wrote in the *Indian Sporting Times*. This was a message that they were eager to hear, since it suggested that British physical superiority wasn't innate.

At the same time, as the Indian independence movement gained strength, Indian nationalists turned away from the accoutrements of the Raj. People who had once worn Western clothes donned garments made from khadi, India's homespun cotton cloth. It's not surprising that they would seek an authentically Indian form of physical culture as well. In hatha yoga—or a modernized, hybrid form of it—they found it. Thus, starting in the nineteenth century, a new, rationalized kind of hatha yoga was born, one that would reach full flower in the twentieth.

~

In the mid-1930s, Eugenia, finally cured of her long malaise, asked a friend of hers, a Nepalese princess named Buba, if she knew where she could find a yoga teacher. Buba referred Eugenia to her brother, Prince Mussoorie, who credited the discipline with transforming him from a heavy and unhealthy child into a lithe and vivacious man. The prince, in turn, directed Eugenia to Swami Kuvalayananda's new yogic health center on Bombay's Charni Road, one of the centers of the hatha yoga renaissance.

Kuvalayananda was a charming, solicitous man with a white walrus moustache and corkscrewing white hair that reached his shoulders. "He reminded me of Einstein because he had the same peculiar look in his large brown eyes: speculative, puzzled and naïve at the same time," Arthur Koestler wrote of him in the 1950s.

A dedicated nationalist and yoga revivalist, Kuvalayananda had been at the forefront of hatha yoga's transformation from a mystical, tantric practice into a modern health regimen. Yoga, he believed, could serve as the basis for an authentically Indian kind of physical culture. Motilal Nehru, Jawaharlal's father, praised Kuvalayananda's work, saying, "He opened out an entirely new field of research and has shown that the different aspects of Yogic Culture Therapy could not only stand the fierce light of modern sciences but are well in advance of all that has so far been discovered in the West." Yoga became proof of Indian greatness.

Born Jagannath Ganesh Gune in 1883, Kuvalayananda became deeply interested in both Indian nationalism and physical culture while a young man at Baroda College. He read the works of Bernarr Macfadden, an American muscleman and publishing tycoon, and studied with Rajratna Manikrao, a revolutionary who developed mass gymnastic drills to prepare young men for the anticolonialist struggle.

Like the Theosophists before him, Kuvalayananda dreamed of melding modern rationalism and ancient wisdom. He wanted to reclaim what he saw as India's indigenous system of exercise, while proving its validity in Western terms. So he began conducting experiments, subjecting yogic claims to unprecedented scientific scrutiny. In 1924 he opened the Kaivalyadhama Ashram in Lonavla, southeast of Bombay, where, with the support of a sympathetic prince, he built a laboratory full of the most up-to-date equipment available.

Eventually, he began to systematize series of poses and other yogic practices, prescribing them like medicine for various ailments. To Gandhi, for example, he recommended saltwater and diluted milk in the morning, followed by an enema, *Savasana* (corpse pose), a modified shoulder stand, and nightly massage.

As a recognized expert on physical education, Kuvalayananda sat on government panels to devise exercise regimens for schools. In these, he combined asanas with calisthenics and moves that were traditionally part of the training program for Indian wrestlers—*dands*, or push-ups, and *surya namaskars*, a flowing series of lunges that today form an essential part of modern hatha yoga classes. These assemblages of yoga poses with Eastern and Western bodybuilding techniques set the precedent for contemporary Western yoga.

Kuvalayananda gave yoga classes at the ashram, though these were gentler and more static, geared toward therapy rather than exercise for adolescents. The demand was so great that in 1932 he expanded to Bombay. There, he began offering courses for women, having become convinced that certain yogic exercises, particularly those focused on the abdomen and pelvic area, could aid childbearing. That's where Eugenia was finally introduced to asana practice.

Arriving at the simple two-story building, she was examined by a doctor. She met briefly with the swami himself, though he didn't teach her; she had to study with the women. She was ushered into a room with a matted floor, where several women in saris were practicing individually. A female instructor showed her how to breathe deeply, to expand her chest and the back of her ribs to take in more oxygen. Then she taught Eugenia three poses: a seated forward bend, the plough, and the shoulder stand. Eugenia, who had never before encountered these basic postures, was mortified to find that she was too stiff to do any of them correctly.

When she returned the next day, she asked a fellow student to lean on her back while she bent forward and tried to touch her toes, but the teacher stopped her—forcing the postures was forbidden. All of them, she said, would come in time. "Which will probably be in my next incarnation!" Eugenia said. For the most part, the classes bored and frustrated her. Except for her mother, Eugenia rarely idolized women. She was still looking for a guru who could excite her devotion the way Krishnamurti had, and this teacher, however well intentioned, was no such figure. Nevertheless, she kept going, and slowly started to make progress.

Then, suddenly, at the start of 1936, the Czech government decided to transfer Jan Strakaty to China, and Eugenia's life in India appeared to be coming to an end. She was sad, but took the news with equanimity, prepared for what she hoped would be a novel adventure. Jo returned to Prague right away, but Eugenia stayed on in India several more months, packing up their household and saying her good-byes. When her May 7 departure date arrived, she remembered how destroyed she'd felt all those years ago when she left Der Blaue Vogel, and she marveled that she wasn't overwhelmed now with a similar heartbreak. Certainly, as she spent her last day in Bombay, she was full of nostalgia, thinking back over her first trip through the country with Krishnamurti, and all the activists, artists, princes, and princesses she'd come to know since. Yet she told herself that she had a pilgrim soul and could find peace anywhere on earth. After a decade in the country, she still knew little of hatha yoga, but perhaps she'd internalized a bit of classical yoga's philosophical detachment.

But just a bit. Soon after arriving in Prague, Eugenia and her mother departed for a trip to the fashionable spa town of Karlsbad. It was a beautiful place, famous for its sulfurous hot springs. Situated in an emerald valley, it boasted promenades, luxury shops, and elegant Baroque and Art Nouveau buildings. People went there to recover from various ailments, but also to socialize and parade around in the latest fashions; such spas were famous for their personal intrigue and social climbing. The 1936 season would be one of the last; in 1938 Karlsbad and the entire region of the Sudetenland were annexed by Nazi Germany. Eugenia was largely unaware of the encroaching peril. Rather than being anxious, she was deathly bored.

Seeking to escape the tedious social whirl, she and Sasha moved to a smaller town, where Eugenia spent her days wandering the forests and regressing into elaborate fantasies about Vava, her adolescent love. Her life was heading in a depressing direction, her chance for autonomy, for individual accomplishments, slowly receding.

Then she received the wedding invitation that would transform everything. The nephew of the powerful, forward-thinking Maharaja of Mysore, whom Eugenia had befriended during her years on India's social circuit, was getting married. Perhaps Eugenia was not as resigned to leaving India as she thought, because given the chance to return, she was elated. It wasn't just that the Mysore Palace was one of the most stimulating and opulent environments in the entire subcontinent, but also that under the Maharaja's patronage there was a yoga *shala*, or school, run by the brilliant, stern, and intense yogi Sri Krishnamacharya.

If she went to the wedding, she'd have the opportunity to meet him. It might be her last chance to find a true yoga master and, more than that, to escape the stultification of a life without ambition. Traditional yoga, of course, is supposed to teach you how to renounce worldly goals, not how to achieve them, but Eugenia had never been bound by tradition.

ANDHI CALLED the Maharaja of Mysore the *rajarishi*, or "saintly king." Cultured and introverted, Maharaja Krishnaraja Wadiyar IV made Mysore the most progressive of India's princely states, kingdoms that existed outside the direct authority of the Raj. The maharaja built universities and hospitals and poured money into public works; his state was the first in India to have electric lights. He also spent lavishly on public buildings and landscaping, creating elegant parks, boulevards, and public squares. The state's capital, Bangalore, was known as the Garden City, but the green, temperate city of Mysore, where the royal family lived, was even lovelier.

Arriving at the Mysore Palace after her depressing interlude in Europe, Eugenia found a timeless fantasia, a gorgeous Indo-Saracenic granite monument of graceful, ornate arches and gilded domes. (It was hard to tell that it was a relatively modern structure, completed in 1912 after the older, wooden palace burned down.) Surrounding it were smaller palaces, intricately carved pyramid-shaped temples, and fragrant gardens. Inside the palace, an endless procession of rooms were decorated with the world's finest materials: ceilings were of Burmese teak or Scottish stained glass, doors were inlaid with ivory, and mosaic floors were paved with ivory and semiprecious stones. Visiting dignitaries were seated on elaborate silver chairs with red velvet cushions. During the annual Dasara festival, the Maharaja rode an elephant in a howdah shaped like a temple and plated with eighty kilograms of gold.

The palace's artistic abundance matched its material splendor. The maharaja was a music lover who played the flute, violin, veena, sitar, saxophone, harmonium, and piano, among other instruments, and awoke daily at 5:00 a.m. to practice them. The palace employed celebrated Indian musicians and a European band with a German conductor. (Examiners from Trinity College of Music in London were brought in to make sure that each Western-style musician was up to the highest standards.) On the seventh day of Dasara, the royal court paid homage to Saraswati, the Hindu goddess of knowledge, learning, and the arts, by worshipping the palace's books and musical instruments.

For all the luxury surrounding him, the maharaja was personally austere and reclusive. He was deeply interested in philosophy and, like Tagore, passionate about encouraging the interchange between East and West. He had traveled widely in Europe and hosted Western intellectuals such as Carl Jung and the British astrophysicist Sir Arthur Stanley Eddington at the palace. The maharaja didn't just want to learn from Europe, though. Like his father, who had funded Vivekananda's sojourn in the United States, he wanted to share India's greatness with the world.

Loving the company of writers, the maharaja invited the peripatetic mystic and author Paul Brunton (originally a German Jew named Raphael Hurst) to live at his palace for several years in the 1930s. Brunton saw Krishnaraja as the sort of philosopher king imagined by Plato in *The Republic*, and wrote that the maharaja had "absorbed the best ancient wisdom of [his] own hemisphere and yet respected the best modern achievements of the Occident."

This attitude extended to the emerging hatha yoga renaissance. In addition to being a dedicated scholar, the maharaja was an avid sportsman, and by the early 1930s, he'd helped turn Mysore into "a pan-Indian hub of physical culture revivalism," in Mark Singleton's words. There was already a history of interest in yoga at the palace. A manual compiled by the maharaja's great-grandfather in the mid-nineteenth century contains illustrations of many yoga poses—it's one of the earliest-known records of an asana practice tradition. The maharaja was eager to develop and popularize this tradition, and to that end, he enlisted a brilliant but indigent and obscure yogi named Tirumalai Krishnamacharya.

Krishnamacharya was a compact, proud man with a face like an eagle's. His head was shaved except for a small tuft that marked him as a Brahmin, and on his forehead he painted vertical white lines signifying his caste. Only five feet two inches tall, he was extraordinarily lithe yet strong—a rare silent newsreel of him taken in 1938, when he was already fifty years old, shows him moving through a series of poses with incredible grace and fluidity. Shirtless in a white dhoti, he practices on a carpet outdoors, beginning with his legs folded in a lotus position but lifted off the ground as he balances on his hands. From there, he leaps back into a pose that looks like upward-facing dog, his tongue thrust out of his mouth and his eyes wide open. He contracts his abdomen, pulling his stomach muscles up until they seem to disappear beneath his protruding ribs. After several breathing exercises, he assumes multiple variations on the shoulder stand and the headstand, exercising perfect control as he repeatedly touches his feet down both in front of him and behind him before picking them back up again.

Even more impressive in the newsreel are the feats of one of his students, his brother-in-law B. K. S. Iyengar, who seems to move in slow motion as he jumps from downward dog into an arm balance with outstretched legs, then bends his elbows back and moves his chest toward the earth, as in the half push-up known as *Chaturanga*. From the backbend known as full wheel, he lifts his legs up into a handstand and then swings them through his arms and into a split. Balanced on his forearms, he bends his back until the soles of his feet rest on the crown of his head.

Some of the poses the two men demonstrate in the newsreel are now part of standard yoga styles, but before Krishnamacharya, they weren't known as asanas at all. He was a modern innovator who, in a strategy common to classical Indian philosophy, worked hard to put the authority of a long, distinguished lineage behind his advances. As Fernando Pagés Ruiz wrote in *Yoga Journal* in 2001, "You may have never heard of him, but Tirumalai Krishnamacharya influenced or perhaps even invented your yoga."

Krishnamacharya has since become a legend, and his biography shrouded in myth. It's known that he was born to a distinguished South Indian Brahmin family in November 1888. His father, a scholar, gave him strict, exacting instruction in the Vedas and other religious texts, waking him at 2:00 a.m. to repeat the religious chants he had to learn by heart.

When he was ten, his father died, and he was sent to Mysore to continue his education at the Parakala Math, the monastery of a school of Vishnu devotees.

At sixteen, according to the tale he told his followers, he was visited by a vision of one of his ancestors, the sage Nathamuni, who told him to journey to the town of Alwar Tirunagari, over three hundred miles away in the neighboring state of Tamil Nadu. Once there, he asked an old man where he might find Nathamuni and was directed to a mango grove by the side of a river. By the time he got there he was so exhausted that he fell unconscious. Either asleep or in a trance, he met Nathamuni, and the sage recited a lost text, *Yoga Rahasya*, or "Secrets of Yoga." Upon awakening, according to the story, Krishnamacharya remembered every word Nathamuni had said and would later cite the *Yoga Rahasya* as the scriptural basis for his revolutionary yoga system.

As a teenager and young adult, Krishnamacharya continued to pursue his religious studies in both Mysore and the holy city of Benares, delving deeply into major religious texts and mastering Sanskrit grammar and several systems of Orthodox Hindu philosophy. These milieus, however, didn't give him much opportunity to develop his interest in hatha yoga. One of his teachers suggested that, if he really wanted to master the practice, he make a pilgrimage to Tibet to find a hermit named Ramamohana Brahmachari.

Now, the cave-dwelling Himalayan master is a common trope in Hindu legends, and no evidence remains of Krishnamacharya's journey. Yet, according to the tale he told his disciples, he found the yogi, a tall man with a long beard and wooden shoes, living in a cave with his wife and three children, and he stayed with them for seven and a half years. Ramamohana Brahmachari instructed him in a lost Nepalese text called the *Yoga Kurunta,* which was rich in information about asana and *pranayama.* Krishnamacharya claimed that, under the yogi's tutelage, he mastered three thousand asanas and learned the kind of extreme physiological self-control that would, in time, allow him (seemingly) to stop his heartbeat. At the end of his apprenticeship, his guru instructed him to go home, get married, and spread the message of yoga throughout society.

Which is what Krishnamacharya did. He turned down an opportunity to lead the Parakala Math, which would have required a vow of celibacy. Instead, in 1925, he married a twelve-year-old girl named Namagiriamma and, forgoing the respect and authority he could have earned with a traditional scholarly vocation, began traveling and lecturing in an effort to popularize hatha yoga. For a time, he supported himself by working on a coffee plantation, a humiliation for a man of his caste and learning. On his days off, he gave sideshow-like strongman demonstrations that he hoped would capture the attention of the masses: stopping cars with his bare hands, lifting objects with his teeth, contorting himself into difficult asanas, and slowing his pulse to simulate death.

Krishnamacharya's commitment to his singular path was rewarded when the Maharaja of Mysore attended one of his lectures and, impressed, invited him to come teach at the palace. Charging Krishnamacharya with developing India's great contribution to the world of physical culture, he gave him a wing of Mysore's Jaganmohan Palace, near the splendid palace where he lived, to open a yoga *shala*, and even sent him to Kuvalayananda's pioneering ashram to learn from his experiments.

At the maharaja's behest, Krishnamacharya traveled the country throughout the early 1930s demonstrating the amazing feats of physiological control that his yoga practice made possible. In 1935 a French cardiologist, Dr. Thérèse Brosse, tested Krishnamacharya's purported ability to stop his heart. Using an electrocardiographic lead, a pneumogram, and a pulse wave recording from the radial artery (in the forearm), she found that, indeed, he was able to make his pulse disappear for several seconds. Later, a team of doctors speculated about how he and other yogis achieved this effect. They concluded that, by tensing the muscles of the abdomen and thorax (the yogic technique, or "lock," known as *udhyana banda*) and closing the vocal folds (what yogis call *jalandhara banda*), Krishnamacharya created an "intra-thoracic pressure" that interfered with the blood's return to the heart. Maybe he couldn't stop his heart, but he could make its beats so slow and soft that they were inaudible, itself an amazing feat.

Well before her trip to the Mysore Palace, Eugenia witnessed one of these displays. Krishnamacharya lay down on the floor, breathed deeply, and his pulse appeared to stop. Spectators were permitted to check it; doctors listened to him with stethoscopes. "I really fail to understand how these yogis can produce such phenomena," said a German doctor. Given that, Eugenia replied, why didn't more people study yoga seriously? "Is it," she asked, "because we Westerners think it is beneath our dignity to acknowledge our ignorance of certain physical laws unknown to us, and therefore prefer to dismiss the Indian teachings as fantastic and obscure?"

In Mysore, Krishnamacharya worked in the same Jaganmohan Palace gymnastics hall as H. Anant Rao, a bodybuilding and gymnastics teacher. Palace records make it clear that his teaching was subsumed under physical education: "The Physical Instruction Class was under Mr. V. D. S. Naidu, and during the latter part of the year Mr. Krishnamachar [*sic*] was appointed to teach the Yogic System of exercises to the Prince."

In addition to the prince, Krishnamacharya was charged with teaching yoga to young boys of the royal Ursu caste, who had far too much animal energy for a deliberate, static practice. Thus Krishnamacharya, working in a milieu of experimentation and dialogue among different physical culture systems, pioneered a dynamic, flowing type of yoga that today is often known as vinyasa, which entails a kind of squat-thrust jump-back between poses.

As Singleton has shown, elements of vinyasa yoga bear an uncanny resemblance to the gymnastics system created by the Danish physical education teacher Niels Bukh. Krishnamacharya undoubtedly came into contact with Bukh's gymnastics, since it was used by the British army and was popular in YMCAs throughout India. In one of Bukh's sequences, for example, the student begins sitting up with legs outstretched, as in the yoga *Dandasana* pose. Then he or she jumps back into a plank pose, balancing on hands and toes while holding the body horizontal, before turning over and balancing on one hand and one foot—yoga's *Vasisthasana* pose. From there, the practitioner moves into what Bukh called "Hand Standing pose," which is identical to downward-facing dog, an upside-down V made while standing on hands and feet. All this is accompanied by deep, rhythmic breathing.

Krishnamacharya also drew on the Mysore Palace's own gymnastic tradition. As N. E. Sjoman demonstrates in his book *The Yoga Tradition of the Mysore Palace*, some of Krishnamacharya's asanas are originally found in a palace gymnastics manual titled *Elements of Gymnastic Exercises, Indian System*. "It is quite clear that the yoga system of the Mysore Palace from Krishnamacariar is another syncretism drawing heavily on the gymnastic text, but presenting it under the name of yoga," writes Sjoman.

None of this is to say that Krishnamacharya was a fraud or a plagiarist. He was, rather, a brilliant synthesizer, a man capable of drawing from everything he had at hand to create something vital and new. His yoga was to gymnastics what Vivekananda's spirituality was to Unitarianism or Bollywood is to Hollywood: a modern Indian art developed in dialogue with the wider world.

Eugenia, in turn, would present this system to a world starved for authenticity as the timeless wisdom of the East. Yet first she had to convince the orthodox Brahmin Krishnamacharya to share his secrets with a woman and a Westerner.

Eugenia was one of thousands of royal guests at the maharaja's nephew's wedding. Because Krishnaraja Wadiyar had no children, the young man was his heir apparent, and his marriage to a teenage princess from central India was a particularly grand occasion. *Life* magazine sent a photographer, and ran a piece with the headline "Heir to $400,000,000 Gets Married in India." Festivities began with an act of clemency, as the maharaja threw open the gates of the central jail and released nearly two hundred prisoners. The wedding ceremony was held in the palace's spectacular octagonal marriage pavilion. Cast-iron pillars painted a rich peacock blue supported a soaring domed ceiling made of stained glass with intricate images of peacocks and floral mandalas, motifs repeated on the mosaic floors. It all "presented a scene of Oriental grandeur," reported the *Times of India*.

The groom arrived on a richly caparisoned elephant, following a majestic procession through the palace grounds accompanied by musicians. The bride entered the pavilion with Brahmins chanting Vedic hymns. The two exchanged garlands of flowers and made offerings to a sacred fire, and representatives from all the surrounding Hindu monasteries came to offer their blessings. Afterward, elaborate feasts and music and dance recitals were held.

Eugenia, however, wasn't interested in any of the celebratory indulgence. Her concern was meeting Krishnamacharya. As soon as she arrived in Mysore, she went to the yoga *shala* uninvited and unannounced and asked to speak to the master. He received her in a large, light-filled room, sitting cross-legged on a carpet. At first he was respectful to his patron's guest, but as soon as he realized she wanted to study at his *shala*, his tone changed. "In my school there

are no women, there are only men, and, among them, none are foreigners," he told her firmly. (The only exceptions he made were for
his female relatives—early on, he taught yoga to his wife, his sister-
in-law, and his two daughters.) Eugenia tried to convince him, but
he wouldn't budge. Finally, he ordered her to leave.

She was terribly disappointed, both by her own failure to become
Krishnamacharya's student, and by his depressing conservatism, so
at odds with the sort of unconventional wisdom she'd expected to
discover. But she was not deterred. She decided to go over his head
and speak directly to the maharaja. The maharaja, of course, was
devoted to spreading the wonders of yoga to the West. Eugenia was
his friend and guest. He ordered Krishnamacharya to teach her.

Even when he wasn't being forced to act against his will, Krishnamacharya was a very difficult man. "Guruji had a frightful
personality," writes B. K. S. Iyengar, the younger brother of Krishnamacharya's wife and, in later years, the guru's most famous disciple. Krishnamacharya's moods were unpredictable, and he could
be violent toward those closest to him. "He would hit us hard on
our backs as if with iron rods," writes Iyengar. "We were unable to
forget the severity of his actions for a long time. My sister also was
not spared from such blows."

Iyengar, who died in 2014 at ninety-five, would eventually become
the most celebrated yoga teacher in the world. Yet in the early 1930s,
he was a sickly, skinny adolescent, enervated from bouts of malaria
and typhoid. "My sisters and sisters-in-law used to say that my head
would hang down on a repulsive body in such a way that they never
touched me on account of my appearance," he writes. He was the
eleventh of thirteen children, and his family, already poor, was
driven close to destitution when his father died shortly before the
boy's ninth birthday. At sixteen, he went to live with his sister and
Krishnamacharya, where he was to help with the housekeeping.

Iyengar enrolled in the maharaja's high school and was one of the
few outside the royal family permitted to attend the two-hour classes

held each afternoon in the yoga *shala*. However, he was weak and stiff, and at first Krishnamacharya largely ignored him.

Then, in 1934, Krishnamacharya's prized pupil ran away, no doubt because of his master's punishing discipline. The maharaja was hosting a YMCA conference at the palace, and Krishnamacharya was supposed to give an asana recital. Needing someone to demonstrate, he recruited Iyengar and demanded that he learn a series of difficult backbends within three days. Terrified of disappointing his fearsome brother-in-law, Iyengar pushed himself into the poses. He was left in excruciating pain and had tremors for months, but he did them correctly and even won a fifty-rupee prize from the maharaja. After that, he often demonstrated for Krishnamacharya's presentations.

Seventy years later, Iyengar had only a vague memory of his first meeting with the European lady who started taking classes at the *shala* in 1938. He was sure that had Krishnamacharya known she'd been an actress, no amount of pressure from the maharaja could have convinced him to instruct her.

Luckily, he was unaware. So, gruff and full of resentment, he acceded to his patron's request and took her on. Assuming her interest in yoga was just a momentary fancy, he figured that if he made things unpleasant enough for her, she'd eventually go away. "Why are you going to complicate your life with such a rigorous discipline?" he asked her. Rigorous discipline, though, was exactly what Eugenia was looking for. She needed something to throw her energy and determination into. Her drifting, aimless, too-easy life was driving her mad.

At first, Krishnamacharya entrusted her lessons to one of his students. "From now on, you will have to submit to a severe diet," he told her. She proudly answered that she'd long been a vegetarian. He told her that wasn't enough. While she was studying at the *shala*, she had to give up all "dead" food, meaning anything preserved or refined: white sugar, white flour, white rice, anything canned. Nor was she allowed to eat any vegetables that grew underground, such as potatoes, carrots, or onions—only plants that "receive the rays of the sun." Eggs were off-limits, as was anything spicy, salty, or sour.

She had to give up tea and coffee, a painful sacrifice. She was even told how to chew her food—instead of swallowing, she was supposed to masticate each bite until it disappeared.

Krishnamacharya's student gave her a strict schedule. She was to wake up before sunrise and perform asanas and meditation, then head to the school for more asana instruction. Dinner had to be two hours before sunset, and she had to be in bed by 9:30, meaning there would be no partaking of the festivities at the palace. She had to bathe in lukewarm water and was forbidden to warm herself in front of a fire. She couldn't travel, meaning she'd be separated from her husband for several months.

She was overwhelmed by it all, and somewhat disappointed. "I imagined that I would be undergoing some sort of mystic and occult training, but I was mainly questioned about the movement of my bowels and the effect of the diet and exercises on my system," she writes. Yet Jo, surprisingly, encouraged her. He had much to do to prepare for the move to Shanghai and was happy to have her in one place while he traveled and then got settled in China. So she dedicated herself to the training, making her way from the palace to the *shala* every day after a frugal breakfast. Weeks went by, and Krishnamacharya started to realize that she was serious. "The European student wasn't so delicate as he thought!" she writes. He developed a grudging respect for her and eventually took over her training.

Because Eugenia was a middle-aged woman and not a wiry, hyperactive boy, the yoga that Krishnamacharya taught her was less aerobic than the system he imparted to Iyengar or K. Pattabhi Jois, another of his protégés who would eventually become a world-famous yoga teacher. Yet many of the poses were the same—a combination of seated postures from classical hatha yoga sources and standing lunges and twists adapted from traditional Indian gymnastics and wrestling exercise regimens as well as from Niels Bukh. She learned to sit in a lotus pose, to bend her back into a bow pose, to support herself with her legs in the air in a shoulder stand. She was terrified to attempt a headstand, but another student, a sixty-six-year-old man, convinced her that if he could do it, she could, too, and within weeks she was balancing easily in the center of the room.

At first, Eugenia found it all exhausting. She felt sluggish and bloated. Krishnamacharya told her that it would take time for the postures to work on her body and normalize the function of her hormones. This notion that yoga improves the working of the endocrine system has since found support among scientists, with studies showing that hatha yoga has a positive effect on blood glucose levels in diabetes patients, on sufferers of thyroid disorders, and on postmenopausal women plagued by hot flashes. No one is entirely sure how this works. Some of yoga's benefits come from the way it combines mindfulness meditation, which is known to calm the nervous system, with the salutary effects of exercise. Additionally, recent research has shown that certain movement patterns "interact reciprocally with cognitive and emotional states . . . Yoga, and other repetitive motion patterns appear to restore and entrain the rhythmicity of biological functions that are often disrupted during periods of stress," in the words of a 2009 journal article. Some speculate that yoga's contractions and contortions physically stimulate the thyroid and pineal glands.

Whatever the mechanism, it worked on Eugenia. As the months passed, the benefits of her new lifestyle began to show. The bloating went away, and she started losing weight. Her skin became smooth and radiant. Naturally, she was elated by the changes. "I felt as light and carefree as a school girl on a summer vacation," she writes. Her depression and anxiety abated. She was grounded and focused as never before.

As part of the second stage of her training, Krishnamacharya initiated her into his methods of *pranayama*, or breath control. He hewed to the traditional view of *pranayama* as a powerful secret that must be learned directly from a master. Locking the door so no one could bother them, he taught her how to breathe through one nostril and then the other and how to retain the breath for various lengths of time. Given all the drama around it, she expressed surprise at how simple it seemed. "He told her that although Pranayama may seem simple, it is extremely powerful and, used wrongly, can be disastrous, leading to 'serious physical and mental troubles.'" There was still a bit of occultism, a bit of dangerous magic, in this yoga. After her own catastrophic attempt at amateur yogic healing, she no doubt took his admonition seriously.

Eugenia's life at the palace and the *shala*, at once luxurious and monastic, continued for eight months, until December, when it was time for her to join her husband in Shanghai. One day, toward the end, Krishnamacharya told her he had plans for her. As her training had gone on, her powerful charm had begun to work on him, and like his patron the maharaja, he'd come to believe that yoga wasn't an art just for Indians, that it should be spread worldwide.

"Now that you are going to visit other countries in the world," he told her, "I want you to teach yoga."

The idea terrified her, and Eugenia protested, saying she couldn't teach what she'd only just learned herself.

"You can do it and you will do it!" he replied firmly.

They spent the time until her departure reviewing her lessons. She'd kept notebooks throughout her stay in Mysore, and together they went over the details of asanas, diet, breath, relaxation, and meditation, with Krishnamacharya explaining how she should impart it all to her future students. She still wasn't sure she'd ever have any, but he was her guru. She couldn't refuse.

PART III

Indra Devi

UGENIA'S SHIP arrived in Shanghai on a cold, damp day toward the end of December 1939. Storm clouds darkened the sky, and the wind whipped her clothes around her legs as her boat steamed up the sludgy Whangpu River to moor off the Bund, Shanghai's great ersatz European boulevard. The city's legendary skyline was a towering wall of gray granite and marble buildings in a potpourri of Western styles, evidence of Shanghai's status as a Far Eastern outpost of both Europe and America. Encountering her new home, Eugenia writes, "I was invaded by a thick, colorless melancholy."

It wasn't just that she missed India. Upon leaving Mysore, she'd spent several months in Bombay before sailing for China. It's not clear why she was delayed there for so long, but she may have put off her trip because she was, once again, in love. In books and interviews, she would sometimes briefly mention a man named Indra Dev, a Dutch aristocrat by birth who had originally come to India to study yoga and classical Indian dance. Despite his youth, Eugenia later said, he was "far advanced along the spiritual path," and he taught her concentration and meditation techniques.

Her descriptions never go further than that, but in later years, she often spoke of him to friends as one of her great romances, though she said it was a spiritual rather than a sexual love. He was, she said, thin and graceful, almost fey—in the one picture she showed to confidants, he had a flower in his dark hair. The name he adopted, so much like hers, was just the beginning of the correspondence between them. Their souls, she said, had merged. (It's possible that it was in homage to him that she would eventually drop the second *i* in her pseudonym Indira Devi.) Yet they couldn't remain together— she had both a husband and a mission in China.

This romance would explain the overwhelming depression that descended on her during her last days in India. "I understood then why people commit suicide, not being able to stand this suffocating agony, which seems to crush the heart like a heavy weight," she writes. It was her old friend and master Krishnamurti who finally jolted her out of her anguish, arriving in Bombay just as she was preparing to leave. At first she went daily to the talks he gave to a study group at the home of an old Theosophist named Ratansi Morarji, but she was so distracted by her own unhappiness that his words barely registered. Finally, during a private meeting with her onetime guru, she confessed her sorrows.

"Do you know what the real cause of your suffering is?" he asked her. "It is fear. You are afraid to face your troubles. In the process of discovering the cause of sorrow, which is craving, you face utter loneliness. You are fully awake only when you are not trying to avoid something, when you are not trying to escape from the inevitable, which is to be alone. And through the ecstasy of that solitude you will realize Truth."

His words, though stern, had a transformative effect on her, breaking through her despondent miasma. They would, in some sense, govern all her relationships going forward—she would never again seek to become one with another person and would cherish her independence above all else. By the time she boarded the ship for China, she felt peaceful, if not exuberant. She had no interest in the social life on the boat, but she attributed this to spiritual development, not depression. While dressing for dinner her first night at sea, she writes, "I discovered that I didn't care any more to decorate myself with jewels and make up my face with lipstick and rouge . . . It felt strange to think that [I] was once a good companion for those who enjoyed gaiety, cinemas, and dancing." She kept to herself, reading, meditating, and helping to nurse a sick old man on board. It's hard to imagine what her husband, Jan, thought of the subdued, sari-clad woman who met him when the ship docked.

If Eugenia was feeling quiet and reserved, her new home was anything but. For Shanghai's newcomers, the sensory assault rivaled that of Bombay. "As you stepped ashore Shanghai's inimitable odour of expensive scent and garlic overwhelmed you," writes one of the city's chroniclers. "A dozen different languages assailed your ear. Beggar children tugged at your clothes. American cars hooted at your rickshaw puller. Trains hurtled past. Above your head the foreign buildings of the Bund thrust into the sky. At your feet Chinese beggars picked at their sores. Down a side street a middle-aged Russian woman and a pubescent Chinese girl fought over a sailor."

Shanghai in the late 1930s was a place where all the players in the incipient Second World War coexisted in an uneasy, unstable equilibrium, and it was thick with intrigue and violence. Among many of the foreigners, a mad, apocalyptic joie de vivre prevailed. In some ways Shanghai, the fifth-largest city in the world and the most cosmopolitan, blended every place Eugenia had ever lived. Cyrillic signs lined Avenue Joffre, an area known as Little Russia. Like Bombay, the city was run by a smug Western colonial establishment unaware of the titanic forces emerging to put an end to its rule. Thousands of eastern European Jews brought a taste of Berlin and Austria to the city, opening restaurants such as Café Louis on Bubbling Well Road, famous for its pastries, handmade chocolates, and sweet Berliner Weisse cocktails, a mix of weak local beer and raspberry syrup. Both its rampant gangsterism and wild nightlife put Weimar to shame. There was even a Berlin-style cabaret, the Black Cat on Roi Albert Avenue, where the famed comedian Herbert Zernik delivered his biting routines.

Shanghai's internationalism was the result of its odd status as a city over which no nation held full sovereignty. The British had made their way into China by force a hundred years earlier, sending a flotilla of gunboats to exact outrageous concessions from the Tao-kuang emperor, including the opening of five Chinese ports to foreign settlement and trade. Shanghai was the most lucrative, and soon other nations demanded a piece of it. What eventually evolved was a city divided into three, each section with its own government and police force. Of Shanghai's twenty square miles, twelve and a half were controlled by foreigners. The British and Americans ruled the International Settlement, where Sikh policemen brought from India patrolled the streets. The French Concession was under the sovereignty of Paris. With some exceptions, Western residents of these enclaves lived outside the jurisdiction of Chinese law, subject instead to courts run by Europeans and Americans. The Chinese had what was left of Shanghai, including the original walled city.

Because of its odd jurisdictional arrangements, Shanghai was a free city—one needed no passport or visa to enter. Thus as war ravaged Europe, huge numbers of the suddenly stateless arrived in Shanghai seeking refuge. The White Russians came first, fleeing the revolution by the tens of thousands, and eventually forming the largest foreign community after the Japanese. There were six daily Russian newspapers; a popular Russian bookstore, Russkoe Delo, with an inventory of fifteen thousand volumes; and a Russian radio station. The shabby elegance of the White Russians played a huge role in the city's expat culture. Most of the big hotels had Russian orchestras and singers. Impoverished masters living in tiny cellar rooms gave music lessons. Former White Russian soldiers earned a living as nightclub bouncers or bodyguards for the warlords who still ruled much of China.

Shanghai's refugee community ballooned still further in the late 1930s as Hitler consolidated power and more than eighteen thousand Jews poured in. The Nazis had allowed them to take only twenty reichsmarks and a suitcase, so they arrived desperately poor. Many quickly set about selling whatever they'd been able to carry out, "everything from handbags and rugs and porcelain to shoelaces," in the words of one Shanghai journalist. "All the moneyed residents of Shanghai went mad for Austrian glassware and china." Some of the Jews were able to raise enough money to rent a room or two and start small businesses. Others crowded into refugee camps at the city's edge.

When Eugenia arrived, many other diplomatic wives, less used to instability than she was, were leaving for what seemed like safer outposts in Hong Kong and Manila. After setting up the puppet state of Manchukuo, in China's north, in 1931, the Japanese had slowly closed in on Shanghai, and in 1937 they seized control of the city's Chinese areas and put them under the control of Chinese puppet rulers. The occupiers waged a terror campaign against their political enemies. Severed heads of Chinese seen as opponents of the Japanese appeared on lampposts around town. American and European journalists were targeted as well; someone threw a grenade at the celebrated correspondent John B. Powell, despite the presence of a bodyguard.

Officially, protections for the international communities in Shanghai remained in place. However, after the defeat of France by Germany in 1940, control of Shanghai's French Concession passed to the Vichy government, which was collaborating with the Nazis. Japan joined the Axis powers in September of that year, making the city's status as a refuge even more fragile. As the American and British colonies shrank, the German presence grew. A Nazi newspaper was printed and sold in the International Settlement.

This was a strange environment in which to open a yoga school, but Eugenia was determined to do as her master had said. At first, when she informed her husband that she would no longer content herself with an "empty social life" and that she intended to work, he was amused and condescending. After all, what did she know how to do? When she told him she planned to teach yoga, he was mortified—for a diplomat in China, "face" was everything. "Do anything you want, but not this nonsense, please," he said. It seemed to him, she writes, just "the crazy idea of an idle society woman, who happened to be his wife."

Jan was already on edge. He was a diplomat of a government that no longer existed. The Nazi Wehrmacht had marched into Czechoslovakia in March 1939. From London, Edvard Beneš, president of the first Czechoslovak Republic, set up a Czech government-in-exile. Strakaty prevailed on the Czech ambassador to China, Jan Seba, not to hand over the embassy to the Germans, but Seba didn't listen. Yet, instead of quitting in protest, Strakaty stayed on, working with the German trade representative, a decision that aroused suspicion among some of his countrymen.

There were several hundred Czechs in Shanghai, and they formed a resistance organization, the Czechoslovak Circle, which rejected all contact and cooperation with Nazi Germany. Strakaty was active in the Circle—by January 1940 he had become its second vice president—but he wavered in his commitment. No one knew how the war was going to go. Unlike the Americans and the British, neither he nor his wife had a country to return to. The destitute refugees filling the city were a reminder of the degradation of dispossession.

Eugenia, like her husband, had an instinct for survival that vied with her idealism. Though she'd had the option of receiving a Soviet passport on account of her Latvian origins, she'd opted instead to get a protectorate passport from the German embassy, which provided her with a modicum of safety. (Jan had kept his Czech passport.) She hated Nazism and was enormously concerned about Shanghai's Jews, but she was also a stateless person, and she saw the direction the war seemed to be moving in.

As he tried to secure his place in this chaotic new world, Strakaty began developing a reputation for unsteadiness and cowardice, qualities he tried to mask with swaggering boasts. "The members of the 'Circle' were mostly brave and unyielding of values, thus showing qualities not found in that crucial era in some indecisive, cautious or fearful people," reads a confidential 1946 memo from the Czech ambassador in China. "Mr. Strakatý appears to belong to the latter category." In the summer of 1939, before Eugenia arrived, he'd already been thrown out of a secret Czech resistance committee (separate from the Circle), which he'd joined in the spring.

Shortly after Eugenia got to Shanghai, Strakaty received an order from Berlin to hand his office directly over to the Germans. He told the Circle he wouldn't do it. Then, it seems, the Germans made him an offer, and on January 18 he capitulated, "without prior notification of the Circle committee, notwithstanding how he used to boast his bravery in the presence of the Committee members," in the words of a postwar Czech government report on the matter. In return, the Germans made him a payment of "several monthly salaries." With the proceeds, he bought a small noodle factory. (A few years later, he expanded into sausage manufacturing, something that didn't much please his strictly vegetarian wife.)

Because of his apparent inconstancy, Strakaty was thrown out of the Czechoslovak Circle. He and Jan Seba tried to create an alternative organization, the Association of Czech and Slovak Residents in China, but it attracted barely enough members to fill its governing committee.

In order not to embarrass her husband further, Eugenia didn't use her married name when she set herself up as a teacher. Sometimes she introduced herself as Regina Petersen. Other times, using the name from her cinema days, she called herself Indira Devi. Occasionally, perhaps in homage to her recently lost love, she shortened the first name to Indra.

Students did not flock to her. Shanghai had a Theosophical Society, and the Russians brought with them their interest in the occult, but hatha yoga was still largely unknown. The first person to call on her wanted to know if she could communicate with spirits. A month after finding space in a gymnasium and starting her new venture, she didn't have a single student. Then someone suggested she put on a conference for people in the diplomatic world, inviting them to learn what yoga actually was. She did, and soon a number of curious American women showed up for class, including Josie Stanton, the American consul's wife. Other people connected to the embassy followed. Devi was invited to give further talks: at the European Medical Association, the Chinese Buddhist Society, the American Community Church, and the Theosophical Lodge. She even presented at the Rotary Club.

Soon her classes outgrew the space she was renting in the gym. At the time, she and her husband were living in hotels, and one of her students found them a flat in the elegant Gascogne apartment building on Avenue Joffre in the French Concession, with the condition that she hold yoga classes there. By day, Devi turned the drawing room into a yoga studio, carefully moving all the furniture back in its place so no trace would be left when Strakaty got home. Soon her beloved mother came to Shanghai to join her, escaping the war in Europe.

When the classes outgrew the apartment, another student arranged for the Strakatys to move into a bungalow on Rue Francis Garnier owned by Madame Chiang Kai-Shek, wife of the Nationalist Party leader Generalissimo Chiang Kai-shek. (At the time, Chiang and his wife were living in Chungking, hundreds of miles to the west, where he had set up a provisional government.) "We did the exercises in Madame's bedroom, which was large enough to hold 25 pupils," Devi recalled years later. She hired a young Russian poet named Michael Volin and his wife, Elena, as assistants, and with their help, she was able to hold up to five classes a day, teaching hundreds of students. (Years later, Volin would become known as the man who brought yoga to Australia.)

None of Devi's classes before the 1960s was recorded, but judging from her books, her system seems to have stayed the same for her first few decades as a teacher. "Before we start on our lesson today, let me greet you, and welcome you to our class," begins a session captured on vinyl, her voice trilling, her crisp words spoken in an indefinable eastern European accent. "I hope you will be a good pupil, and that yoga postures will do to you what you expect them to do to you."

She began by having her students practice deep, rhythmic breathing, urging them to sit up straighter and to use the back of the throat to push air in and out. "Very relaxed! Not being stiff," she commanded. She led her class through a number of respiration exercises. They began lying down, breathing in and out to slow counts of four. Then they stood up, inhaled, and held their breath before exhaling, as she commanded, "with great force. Out all the impurities. Especially people who smoke!"

After that came neck rolls and stretches, eye exercises, and "sound vibrations" (one or two syllables held as long as possible). As was her fashion, she explained the efficacy of this chanting in empirical terms: "Very few people realize the importance and the potency of the vibrations that we can produce by our voice, because it gives like an inner massage to the entire body, our glands, our organs are getting the benefit of these inner vibrations." The class began with "eeeeeeeaaaaahhhhh," then proceeded to "aaaaaaaaeeewwww," and finally the familiar "oooohhmmmm."

Unlike most contemporary teachers, she led her students through deep relaxation before starting them on asanas, having them lie on their backs and systemically let go of tension in each part of the body, beginning with the toes. "Imagine for a while . . . that you are a cloud," she said. "Very light, very relaxed, just floating in the sky, passing by another cloud, and gently gliding along, over a green valley . . . over a lake in which you can see your reflection like in a mirror." She told them to keep out all thoughts of their lives and let themselves sink into nothingness, and then to start breathing in "vital cosmic energy."

Only after twenty or so minutes of preliminaries did the asanas begin. As she led her students from a bridge into a shoulder stand—she called it "the reverse posture—she explained that the latter was a "youth-giving posture. It has an effect on our thyroid glands and on our sex glands, and because of that it is supposed to banish premature wrinkles, give vitality, and keep us in a youthful condition much more than you would expect." She took her students through gentle backbends (cobra and locust, or *Salabhasana*), explaining the promised physical benefits as she went. She had them attempt lotus pose and then bend forward, foreheads on the floor, which she said would help to keep the intestinal tract clean.

"In the more advanced stages of yoga, this posture is helping us to develop our spiritual qualities, because it helps to awaken our *kundalini*, our dormant powers," she said. "But in the first stage, it will just help you to keep in good health." She was a big believer in the power of the headstand, using a wall to help novice students get upside down. The classes weren't vigorous, but they were challenging, particularly for those with tight hips, who had a hard time folding their legs into lotus pose.

Most of Eugenia's pupils were Americans. A customs official in his fifties became a convert after six weeks of yoga eased the headaches that had plagued him all his life. Another student, a thin woman whom Devi called "Mrs. B.," was wracked with insomnia and anxiety that made her nearly suicidal. After six months of classes, Devi writes, she "looked the picture of health . . . and swore she would not touch medicines any more." Eugenia gave lessons to a young Chinese boy suffering from asthma who, after two months, brought her a huge bouquet of flowers from his grateful parents.

Eugenia moved easily among the eccentric remnant of Shanghai's expat society. The American military attaché remembered her as one of the few White Russians who was fully accepted by the American colony, which sometimes led to envy among her countrymen. She certainly didn't share the White Russians' customary prejudices, throwing herself into fund-raising for the city's Jewish refugees. Occasionally, over Jan's embarrassed objections, she'd give benefit performances of dances she'd learned in Bombay. "I don't know anything about India but I thought she danced awfully well," writes journalist Emily Hahn.

Hahn, who went by the nickname Mickey, was one of Shanghai's most intriguing characters. A beautiful Jewish woman from St. Louis with dark bobbed hair and wry almond eyes, she shared Eugenia's intrepid spirit, if not her spiritual longings. Hahn had worked as a horseback guide in New Mexico in the 1920s and traveled through Central Africa on her own in the 1930s, serving for a while at a medical clinic in the Belgian Congo reachable only by boat. She'd ended up in Shanghai somewhat by accident, after taking a trip to the Orient with her sister to distract herself after a failed romance with the Hollywood screenwriter Eddie Mayer. She fell in love with China and stayed, publishing dispatches and autobiographical short stories in *The New Yorker* and other publications.

Hahn had a number of dalliances, among them with the extravagantly wealthy businessman Sir Ellice Victor Sassoon, part of a family of Baghdadi Jews known as the Rothschilds of the East. He gave her a shiny blue Chevrolet coupe that she drove to get out of the city on weekends. The man Hahn was closest to, though, was Sinmay Zau, an elegant, irreverent, and married Chinese poet. He was the one who introduced her to opium, a vice on which, for a time, she was dependent.

It was a shocking thing, in Shanghai's colonialist expat culture, for an American woman to take a Chinese lover. Hahn didn't care. She enjoyed her scandalous, exotic image. Having fallen in love with apes in Africa, she bought herself a pet gibbon that she named Mr. Mills. Beige with a black face, Mr. Mills stood about a foot and a half tall. Hahn took him everywhere, often perched on her shoulder. When she went to dinner parties, she dressed him up in a diaper and fur suit made of trimmings from her sable coat. Later, she added old, sick Mrs. Mills to the household—the sight of the pitiful ape in a pet shop had been too heartbreaking for her to resist.

Hahn and Eugenia became fast friends. They met when Eugenia was seeking Indian musicians for one of her performances and someone sent her to Hahn, who knew everyone. (One of Hahn's suitors was there that day and suggested that Eugenia look among the Indian policemen, which she ended up doing.) After that, Eugenia often called on Hahn. "She was an eccentric person, fond of refugees, Yogi, India and Indian dances—any number of disassociated interests," Hahn writes. Eugenia had introduced herself as Regina Petersen, and Hahn called her Peter.

Not all Hahn's friends appreciated her primates. One Englishwoman enraged the journalist by inviting her to a party but writing on the invitation, "Sorry we cannot extend invitation to Mr. Mills." Eugenia, however, adored them. Hahn recalled, "Once when Peter . . . dashed in and kissed me, Mrs. Mills bit her savagely, sink-ing her tusks in up to the gums. I was scared to death, but Peter as a gibbon lover refused to complain."

Like Hahn, Eugenia tended to her image. Since studying with Krishnamacharya, she'd committed herself to monthly days of silence, a practice she kept up for the rest of her life. Still, rather than stay home in quiet meditation, she went out and about in the city, "shaking her head and placing her finger to her lips mysteriously if some uninitiated person spoke to her," writes Hahn.

These days of silence drove Eugenia's husband mad; he accused her of mindlessly imitating Gandhi and told their friends that if she could, she'd go about in a loincloth. Yet Hahn and her lover found Eugenia's quirks delightful. "Sinmay adored her in his own way; she appealed to his love of the bizarre," Hahn writes. "He could sit and watch her for hours, smiling to himself, now and then asking a question guaranteed to send her pelting off in pursuit of one of her hobbies."

Hahn had little patience, however, for Eugenia's attempts to enlist her in her schemes to help Shanghai's Jewish refugees, an issue that already consumed Hahn. "I was spending ninety per cent of my time on them anyway," she writes. "Peter added the missing ten per cent to my program." When Hahn protested, Eugenia just laughed and gave her an affectionate pat on the cheek. Once, Eugenia brought a young Jewish writer named Mr. Levin to Hahn's home, hoping the journalist could help him. Hahn was tremendously irritated—so much so, in fact, that she realized she was becoming completely burned out. "Mr. Levin's image pursued me; I could not shake it off my mind," she writes. "His silly, self-eager face, his boyish prattle, summed up for me all of demanding humanity. It seemed to me suddenly that all the clocks in Shanghai were ticking fast and faster, and my heart beat slow and slower." She wanted to leave town, but the Japanese occupation made travel difficult. So she withdrew for a while, asking her servants to tell all visitors that she wasn't at home.

A little later, Hahn sailed for Hong Kong to finish the book she was writing about Madame Chiang Kai-shek and her influential sisters. She expected to return in three months. "Probably in the back of our heads was the thought, 'The really grim things, the big bomb-ings and battles, never come out as far as the East. We fought the war at long distance last time and we'll fight it like that again,'" she writes. She never saw Shanghai again.

One day on Avenue Joffre, Eugenia passed a Russian restaurant named after Alexander Vertinsky, the cabaret singer she'd last seen in Ukraine. Curious, she stepped inside, and soon heard, "Zhenia! It can't be!" Before her was the friend with whom she'd once traveled snowy streets by troika as he pursued the beautiful Valentina Sanina. After the war, Vertinsky had followed the White Russian emigra-tion to Istanbul, where he opened the Black Rose cabaret. When the Russians started leaving Turkey, he went to Paris, before settling in Hollywood, where he reportedly had an affair with Marlene Die-trich. The Great Depression sent him abroad once again, and he had ended up in Shanghai.

It wasn't an entirely comfortable reunion. Eugenia had little inter-est in joining the White Russian laments for the lost czarist empire. Constantly propelling herself forward, she was masterful at moving on. Her refusal to look back began as a survival strategy and, as she studied yogic ideas of detachment, became a spiritual principle. She was allergic to nostalgia. Vertinsky wasn't; he longed for Russia. Not long after their meeting, unable to bear his homesickness, he decided to return to the Soviet Union. Because Stalin was a devoted fan, Ver-tinsky was able to resume his celebrated career on the Russian stage.

There was only one Russian in Shanghai with whom Eugenia became deeply close: the Jewish composer Aaron Avshalomov, a slight but handsome man with hooded, haunted eyes and wavy gray hair that swooped up from his high forehead. Born in Siberia, Avsh-alomov was five years older than Eugenia. Like her, he'd grown up convinced his destiny lay eastward and had led an equally itinerant life, one that, as time went on, he dreamed of joining with that of the woman he called "the Indian dancer."

Avshalomov fell in love with Chinese music and theater as a boy, when one of his father's employees, a man from Shandong Province named Tung Fa, amused him by banging a gong, walking on stilts, and dressing up like a Han Dynasty warrior and performing war dances. After contracting pneumonia during a brief stint in the army during World War I, Avshalomov moved to Tientsin, a treaty port in northern China, where he found work playing the violin in a hotel. He earned enough to buy a steerage ticket to America, lived for a while in San Francisco, and married a woman named Esther. In 1917 he returned to China, dreaming of composing music that combined Western orchestration with Chinese motifs and melodies. He wrote a Chinese opera, *Kuan Yin*, the name of the Buddhist goddess of mercy, then returned to the United States for a couple of years. By 1929 he was back in Tientsin with his wife and young son, Jacob.

Eventually Avshalomov moved to Shanghai, where he took a job as Shanghai municipal council librarian while he continued to pursue his music. He also took a lover, Tatiana, an earthy, saucy woman who believed herself something of a clairvoyant. Avshalomov moved in with her and her young son, Victor, while Esther and Jacob remained in Tientsin. He found increasing success with his music; in 1935 his symphonic sketch *Hutungs of Peking* was performed by the Philadelphia Orchestra, conducted by the famous Leopold Stokowski.

When Avshalomov met Eugenia, he was in the middle of a long, drawn-out divorce from Esther, who had charged him with bigamy for his relationship with Tatiana. This didn't dissuade him from his new infatuation. Unlike Eugenia, Avshalomov had a tendency toward self-pity and despair. "I feel old and tired, not so much in body as in spirit," he wrote to his son in April 1939. "This waiting, always waiting for something to happen, saps my energy . . . It is only by force of habit that I write at all, a few bars a day, and not every day." By May, however, his letters appeared more cheerful, and he mentioned, for the first time, "a dancer of Indian dances."

Avshalomov was so taken with Eugenia that he began composing Indian-themed music for her. In a July letter to his son, he wrote of "rehearsing the Indian dances with Indira Devi about whom I wrote some time ago. She is a wonderful inspiration." The pieces were performed twice, in Jessfield Park, a popular outdoor performance venue, and then again in French Park, with the Italian maestro Mario Paci conducting. "Indira Devi danced exceptionally well, and every movement of her expressive gestures corresponded to the rhythms and phrases I conceived," raved the besotted composer. In another letter, he tried to justify betraying Tatiana, whom everyone called Tanya, for Eugenia. "Creative work will always require new stimulus which no one woman can sustain," he wrote.

It's hard to say how Eugenia saw all this, since she never mentions Avshalomov in any of her published writing. One of her students, the secretary to the U.S. military attaché, said that though Eugenia saw herself and the composer as "kindred souls," their relationship was platonic. As Eugenia was married, it surely behooved her to give that impression, but while she probably wasn't ever in love with Avshalomov, theirs was more than simply a devoted friendship. It's not surprising that Tanya hated her and objected to her and Avshalomov's collaborations. "The ballet has again twice been given up for dead," Avshalomov lamented in 1941. "First time on account of my collaboration with Indira Devi . . . leading to such drama that I decided to give up on it."

As their small drama played out, a larger and far more serious one was going on all around them. Day by day, Shanghai life grew more unsettled as the Japanese grip on the city tightened inexorably. There was a frenetic surface jollity—"To get into a movie on a week-end without an advance booking was out of the question," writes journalist Vanya Oakes, a friend of both Eugenia and Avshalomov. "The night clubs, overflowing with champagne, were packed." Business and finance proceeded at their usual headlong pace. "But underneath[,] Shanghai was already suffering from a creeping, miasmic fever and there was the ominous gathering confusion of a household where someone is falling very sick indeed," Oakes writes. Law and order broke down further. Within the once-safe International Settlement, drivers were held up at gunpoint. "Shanghai," says Oakes, "had become a city where there might easily be a corpse on the side-

walk on Saturday which would still be there on Monday." But neither Eugenia nor Avshalomov had anyplace else to go.

At 4:30 in the morning on December 8, 1941, Shanghailanders
awoke to the sound of explosions. John Potter, an American businessman, was staying at the Shanghai Club on the Bund, and he
rushed to his window. "There on the river stretch just before the club
was a vivid scene of war," he recalled, writing of the streaks of tracer
bullets that "chased one another in low curves. Then came bursts of
flame from the target." That was the British warship *Petrel*, which
Japanese boats had attacked. As it burned, billows of black smoke
obscured the sky.

At the same time, Japanese solders occupied the American gun-
boat *Wake*, arresting and imprisoning its crew and replacing the
Stars and Stripes with the Rising Sun. In the city, diplomats from
Allied countries were rounded up and put under house arrest at the
Cathay Mansions, a luxury apartment building in the French Con-
cession. Japanese columns poured into the international settlement.
All the city's British and American troops had left to fight the war
elsewhere. Now the war had finally come to Shanghai.

"The Imperial Japanese Army and Navy declare that a state of
war exists between the Imperial Government of Japan and the Gov-
ernments of Great Britain, the United States of America, and the
Netherlands," read proclamations plastered all over the International
Settlement. "All people must proceed with their business as usual,
and the Japanese will protect friends and enemies alike."

By midday, American government offices had been seized, and
officials and staff were interned at the Metropole Hotel. Among
them were some of Eugenia's students and her students' husbands.
The hotel wasn't sealed off, and dazed members of the American
community gathered in the Art Deco building, crowding around
radios, where reports of the Japanese bombing of Pearl Harbor were
being broadcast by shortwave from San Francisco.

Eugenia made her way there through the afternoon drizzle. On the streets, things seemed weirdly normal. Trams and buses ran, and restaurants and department stores were open. At the hotel, finding friends and students captive and anxious, she did the only thing she could think of to help—she led them through a yoga class. "I shall never forget . . . the unique experience of conducting an unusual 'prison class,' which comprised the entire staff of the American Consulate that was kept under arrest in the Metropole Hotel," she writes.

Perhaps on account of her German papers, the Japanese guards let her come back in the following weeks to teach again. She had to keep her distance from the students, who gathered in a semicircle on the blue carpet of the hotel's former dining room, "with a Japanese sentry at the door to prevent any message-carrying or private conversations." Years later, some of these students would tell her how much yoga had helped them during the ordeals that followed.

In the first days after the Japanese takeover, a strangely exciting sort of solidarity settled over Shanghai's international community. One woman recalled going to the bank a few days after the occupation began—it was opened for two hours only, and was allowing people to withdraw only five hundred dollars at a time. "Stood for 1½ hours in the queue, but it was not hardship, nice and sunny, immense friendliness and community of spirit from everybody, but why does it need a catastrophe to produce a condition which ought to be as natural to humanity as breathing?" she writes. There was great hope that once the United States joined the war, it would quickly come to an end. "We could hardly foresee a war of several long years," recalled Potter.

But over the coming weeks and months, life in Shanghai quickly deteriorated. American, British, and Dutch businesses were seized. A proclamation ordered all citizens of Allied countries to register at the Enemy Aliens Office at Hamilton House, a commandeered apartment building in the International Settlement. Each enemy national was given a bright red armband marked with a *B* for British, *A* for American, *N* for the Netherlands, and *X* for smaller countries such as Greece. (Indians and other Asians who fell under the sovereignty of these nations were excepted.) The red armbands had to be worn in public at all times, and those sporting them were barred from theaters, cabarets, and restaurants with music.

The Japanese froze enemy nationals' bank accounts, allowing them to withdraw only two thousand Chinese dollars a month, forcing people used to living in colonial luxury to survive on the budget of a lower-middle-class Chinese family. Cars without Japanese plates were barred from the roads. People accustomed to chauffeured sedans took to riding bicycles. Those who could afford them started using horses and carriages; one famous Polish dressmaker attached a coachman's seat to her glossy blue sedan.

Inflation went wild, and because all commerce passed first through Japanese hands, staples began disappearing from shops. Once again, Eugenia was in a city where formerly comfortable people, suddenly destitute and bewildered, had to queue for hours to buy meager rations. Of course, for most Chinese people, things were far worse. Often they'd start lining up to buy rice off incoming ships the night before. "Hundreds of Chinese dead were picked up on the streets each morning, victims of hunger and exposure," writes one resident.

Because of their German and Czech papers, Eugenia and her husband were better situated than many of her friends. They continued to live comfortably; indeed, businessmen such as Jan Strakaty thrived because so many of their former competitors were dispossessed. For those with money, there was food to be had on the black market. Sasha continued to live with them; Russians were closely supervised but remained free. Indeed, writes one historian, "The Russian community enjoyed good amateur theater, dramatic societies, concerts, dancing schools, and ballet performances throughout the war."

Still, there was no escaping the pervasive terror on the streets. People of all nationalities began to disappear, some to the notorious torture chambers at Bridge House, an apartment building turned prison. (After the war, one of Eugenia's students would tell her how much his ability to sit in lotus pose helped him when he was crowded into one of Bridge House's packed and fetid cells.) Everyone lived in dread of an early morning visit from the Japanese gendarmerie. Eugenia was called in for questioning several times, though never detained. She tried to maintain control of Madame Chiang Kai-shek's bungalow by flying the flag of neutral Sweden, her father's country, over it, but was eventually ordered out.

She continued giving classes at home for a while, but soon there was hardly anyone to give classes to. As life grew harder, she and Avshalomov grew closer. To stay sane, he threw himself into work, writing up to fifteen hours a day; during the winter, he scratched out notes with freezing hands while wrapped in blankets. The Westerners left in Shanghai staged musical performances in one another's houses.

Then Avshalomov lost his. In 1943, in a terrifying echo of the slaughter in Europe, most of the Jews who'd arrived in Shanghai from Germany and eastern Europe were ordered into a ghetto in Hongkew, a rundown district across from the International Settlement where they were forced to crowd into squalid tenements. Avshalomov left only scattered notes from this period, but he mentions being put under house arrest on the outskirts of the city. One has to assume that Eugenia visited him there, because by the time the war was over, he trusted her more than anyone on earth.

While conditions in the Hongkew ghetto were dire, they didn't compare to what the Jews of Europe faced. Heinrich Himmler pressured his Japanese allies to begin exterminating the Jews, but the Japanese balked. In fact, the Japanese ended up treating the stateless Jews better than they treated the Americans, British, and Dutch, who were rounded up and sent to internment camps.

The imprisonments began on February 1, with around four hundred young British and American men. Then another seven hundred were called. Over the next four months, all Allied citizens in Shanghai were sent to camps. They were allowed to bring as much as they could carry. "On certain days throughout January and February, anyone walking between the Anglican Holy Trinity Cathedral on Kiangse Road and the tenders on the Bund just before the Soochow Creek would witness the astonishing sight of several hundred white men, women, and children bent under luggage and bedding like proverbial beasts of burden as they made their way from the cathedral toward the boats that would take them to their new homes," writes author Stella Dong.

Some industrious camp inmates organized makeshift universities to keep themselves productive. At Pootung Camp, one could study languages, mathematics, zoology, psychology—and yoga. The last was almost certainly taught by one of Eugenia's students. She would later hear about several such concentration camp yoga classes.

Outside the camps, life was easier but not easy. Ordinary Chinese families were reduced to begging in the garbage-strewn streets. Imperious Japanese soldiers kept the population under tight control and could commandeer property at any moment. Time and again, they'd search Eugenia and Jo's house without any pretext. Eventually, when a Japanese general cast his eye on their home, she, Jan, and Sasha were forced to move, although Eugenia, characteristically bold, refused to leave until the Japanese found them another minimally acceptable place to live. They were fortunate that Jan owned a noodle factory, because many shops had bare shelves.

By the fall of 1944, American air raids had begun. The sight of silver bombers and fighter planes thrilled many desperate onlookers—"it was almost like a fairy tale over Shanghai," said one Russian resident. Still, the bombs and the constant screaming of air-raid sirens were terrifying. The Japanese ordered residents to dig trenches in the streets and imposed a dusk-to-dawn curfew. News was heavily censored, so at night, people huddled around contraband radios, frantic for word of Allied progress. Eugenia thought they were doomed "to be either level-bombed or blown up by the Japanese, who had decided to turn Shanghai into ashes should they lose the battle for it."

She would later write that yoga gave her serenity and equanimity during these years. Still, she thought a lot about death. She began to frequent a Buddhist temple and befriended a young monk there.

One day, she told Jan that should she be killed, she wanted a Buddhist cremation rather than a Christian burial. As usual, he scoffed, telling her that, by law, she had to be buried according to the rites of her legal religion. She wasn't sure he was telling the truth, but just in case, she went to the temple and officially converted to Buddhism, received a document, and gave it to her husband. She never really identified as a Buddhist, but like her yoga practice, which she maintained throughout the bombing, her conversion gave her some sense of control over her own future, ensuring, at the very least, that she'd never be trapped in a coffin.

In the spring of 1945, secret shortwave radios brought news of Hitler's suicide and the Allied victory in Europe. The war in the Pacific dragged on, but the sight of ever more Allied planes in the skies over Shanghai heartened residents. Finally, on August 16, 1945, ten days after an atomic bomb obliterated Hiroshima, Shanghai learned that the war was over. All over the city, radios and loudspeakers played a recording of the capitulation speech that Japanese emperor Hirohito had delivered the day before. Speaking of the "new and most cruel bomb," deployed by the Americans, he said, "[s]hould we continue to fight, it would not only result in an ultimate collapse and obliteration of the Japanese nation, but also it would lead to the total extinction of human civilization."

The whole city poured into the streets, dancing and embracing. Music seemed to come from everywhere, along with the flashing and popping of firecrackers. After years of nightly blackouts, the suddenly lit-up city looked radiant, magical. "Wherever we went, people were crowding and singing, swinging placards and signs; ornaments hung down from lamp posts and wires, flags of the victorious nations waved in the wind, and the entire population was in a most jubilant state," recalled a Jewish man suddenly free from the Hongkew ghetto.

By September, Chinese troops were in control of Shanghai, the port was open, and American firms were once again opening their doors. "Shanghai is now absolutely mad: prices jumping up, cafes, cabarets, bars, girls—all for the military," writes Avshalomov. "It is a gay life for those who have U.S. currency. For the rest—heavy burden and hardships." Thanks to their factory, Eugenia and Jan had access to American dollars. She got rid of her German papers and obtained a Czech passport. Soon she was teaching yoga again.

It's a measure of how quickly the city's social life revived that before the end of the year, Eugenia decided to put on another dance performance, this one to benefit victims of the famine ravaging the Indian state of Bengal. K. P. S. Menon, India's representative to the provisional Chinese government in Chungking, traveled to Shanghai to attend. He'd been delighted, upon meeting her earlier, to realize they had a number of mutual friends. "I was interested to see in her possession a photograph of the youngest Rajkumari of Mysore, for whose marriage to the Maharaja of Bharatpur I was primarily responsible," he wrote in a letter to a British colleague.

After he saw her dance, though, his assessment was vicious. "Indira Devi's much-advertised performance turned out to be a flop," he wrote to another diplomat. "It brought in a lot of money for the Indian Relief Fund but the performance itself was disappointing. It was so amateurish. Her 'mudras' were stiff and artificial and her feet seemed to have no life in them. Moreover she is getting a little too old for the stage. She is 46; and all her yoga practice cannot conceal her age . . . I feel sorry that the first exponent of Indian dancing in Shanghai should have been so poor."

Menon may have been unkind, but he was still worth knowing. By the end of the war, Eugenia's marriage to Strakaty was essentially over, and she began to feel that her relationship with Avshalomov was holding both of them back. With Menon's intercession, she got a visa to travel to India, and in March 1946 she slipped out of town, heading for Bombay aboard the *Highland Chieftain*. She wrote to Avshalomov's son from the ship, "I firmly believe that his star will shoot up soon—only it will not be given me to witness. This is one of the reasons for my speedy departure. Hope he will realize it one day." A few months later, Strakaty, to whom she was still officially wed, sailed home on a British repatriation ship. She'd never see him again.

UGENIA ARRIVED in Bombay in 1946 as the British, exhausted by World War II, prepared to depart. There were furious negotiations about the future of the subcontinent, with Muslim nationalists agitating to carve out an independent Pakistan. Communal violence flared all over the country. British expatriates rushed to pack up their belongings, selling whatever they couldn't take, before independence was declared in 1947.

Eugenia's plan to continue her yoga studies in such conditions wasn't entirely impractical. Yoga was, after all, the one constant in her life, the thing she could turn to whenever everything else crumbled. The new Indian nation would need a new health system, and there was tremendous enthusiasm among Indian leaders to make yoga a part of it. One of Eugenia's friends, Dr. G. V. Deshmukh, a prominent nationalist and a great champion of women's rights, urged her to write a book to help popularize the discipline. He even promised to write the foreword. Other friends, the maharaja and majarani of Tehri Garhwal, offered to host her at their palace in the Himalayas while she worked.

The palace—which today houses the Ananda Spa, perhaps the most sumptuous hotel in India—sits on a ridge overlooking the deep green Doon Valley and, in the distance, the holy city of Rishikesh, situated just over twelve miles away, on the banks of the Ganges. Mircea Eliade once called Rishikesh "the paradise of hermits and contemplatives." Its streets were full of wandering sadhus in saffron robes, naked ash-smeared yogis with dreadlocks piled on their heads like bird's nests, and all manner of monks, swamis, and pilgrims.

Among all these holy men, Eugenia was told, was a yogi so advanced in his practice that he had reached the transcendent state of *samadhi*, the culmination of the yogic journey. Another royal friend of hers, the Rani Madhvi of the princely state of Jasdan, offered her a letter of introduction to the holy man. So she made her way to his Rishikesh ashram, hoping to continue her yogic studies with him while she worked on her book.

In interviews and memoirs, Eugenia never identifies the swami, calling him by the pseudonym Swami Somnatashram. It's extremely likely, however, that it was Swami Sivananda Saraswati, an English-speaking Brahmin physician from Tamil Nadu who, in the 1920s, renounced his comfortable, prosperous life to become a sannyasin in Rishikesh. Like Eugenia's pseudonymous sage, Swami Sivananda was deeply influenced by Vivekananda; he presented yoga as a universal science of life that united the truths of all great religions. In 1936 he founded the Divine Life Society, an organization to propagate yoga and Vedanta. Among its aims was the promotion of healthy living through classes on yoga asanas, breathing, "well-regulated diet . . . well-disciplined life, nature-cure methods."

Even as a mystic, Sivananda injected a strong element of middle-class uplift in his teachings. "His approach to solving the world's problems, as well as India's, was fundamentally grounded in personal reform, both physical and spiritual, and the notion that if each individual made him- or herself into a better person, the world would . . . be a better place," writes scholar Sarah Strauss. The Divine Life Society ashram was deliberately as much a spiritual tourist destination as a traditional hermitage. Sivananda once described it as "an ideal place of retreat for the educated citizen of the world, wherein he can renew himself and recreate and refresh his being, physically, mentally, morally and spiritually." It had, among its supporters, a number of local aristocrats, among them Eugenia's friends.

An imposing, broad-shouldered man with a shiny bald head, Swami Sivananda could be terse and elliptical, frustrating those who came to him in search of clear guidance. When Eugenia sought him out, he told her he wasn't interested in becoming her teacher—he was busy translating ancient manuscripts and had no time for new disciples. Nevertheless, she kept showing up at his ashram in order to be in his presence as he worked. Occasionally, she writes, he would toss off a pithy observation, and she would eagerly latch onto it, feeling like a dog grateful for scraps.

Meanwhile, she struggled with her book, writing draft after draft as she tried to communicate what she'd learned from Krishnamacharya years ago. Her surroundings helped compensate for the pain. In the mornings, she would meditate in one of the palace's shady gardens, listening to the whisper of a small fountain. The maharani had assigned her a servant, and during the afternoons, he would drive her to the temple-filled city, which pulsed with the prayers of wandering holy men, or to the Divine Life Society ashram.

Eventually the swami got used to Eugenia's presence at the ashram and, like Krishnamacharya before him, developed a tolerant affection for her. One day he asked her if she'd yet found a teacher. When she replied that she hadn't, he replied, "Come tomorrow and study with me."

Like Vivekananda, Swami Sivananda divided yoga into four paths: raja, or "kingly," yoga, the yoga of concentration and physical and mental discipline; bhakti yoga, the yoga of devotion; jnana yoga, the yoga of learning; and karma yoga, the yoga of selfless service. Raja yoga, Eugenia writes, was what she learned from her pseudonymous swami. Three times a week she would go to the ashram to study various techniques of sensory withdrawal, concentration, and meditation. Back at the castle, she would try to practice them.

At times, the intense mental discipline was wearying. Vivekananda had warned in his book *Raja Yoga* that before one mastered the practice of concentration, there could be "[g]rief, mental distress, tremor of the body, irregular breathing." Eugenia, who had begun to think of him as a sort of spirit guide, was finding out what he meant. Once, when she was at her desk writing, she had the sense that the room was suddenly full of a dark and fearsome presence. Feeling almost unable to move, she went to bed and lay in a cold sweat. A materialist might interpret what happened to her as a panic attack, not unlike the ones that first drove her to seek relief in yoga. Her teacher told her that sinister forces sometimes arose to impede the spiritual progress of yogis and that she was thus waging a struggle for her soul. That's how she chose to understand it.

In the end, she won. The fear lifted, and she felt calm, buoyant, and productive. She finished her book, *Yoga: The Technique of Health and Happiness*, dedicating it to the "women of India in the person of my gentle and understanding friend without whose encouragement and care this book would not have been written," a reference to the maharani whose palace she was living in. As promised, Dr. Deshmukh wrote a brief foreword. The book itself was divided into two parts: a short, selective autobiography about the role of yoga in her own life, and some practical instruction in asana and diet.

Far from a mystical work, the book argues that modern doctors and scientists had simply discovered what the yogis knew all along about mental and physical hygiene. "People are coming to realize that this system perfected centuries ago, deals in a very thorough way with nerves and glands and their effect on the body," she wrote, promising that the practice would provide "better sleep, a clearer and calmer mind, and a happier outlook on life."

The book pleads with Indians to rediscover the greatness of their own spiritual traditions rather than "blindly copying the West, which is in a state of spiritual and moral bankruptcy and despair. Of late the Occident has been turning its attention to India in the hope of getting some spiritual food, without which men cannot exist for long, however healthy, rich and comfortable they may be." Such sentiments would have been welcome in a country proud of its new independence, though by the time it was published, she'd be gone.

When her writing was finished, Eugenia made plans to teach yoga at a nature cure center that the Cambodian monk Bellong Maha-thera (known as "Bhante" by his legions of admirers) was planning to open in Kashmir. A former judge who'd been educated at the Sorbonne before becoming a wandering forest ascetic, Bhante devel-oped a form of alternative medicine based on vegetarianism and color therapy. He was close to both Gandhi and Nehru; the latter gave him a former Mughal pleasure garden as thanks for curing one of his parents, and turned it into a Buddhist mission. Bhante's ideas about healing meshed with Eugenia's—he believed that many ills could be cured by sunshine, fresh food, and positive thoughts. (He would live to be 110.) Yet before she could start working with him, she received a telegram calling her back to China.

After World War II, Eugenia's mother had stayed behind in their house in Shanghai, happy to live as part of the White Russian community. But while the Japanese occupation was over, China's instability wasn't. The civil war between China's Nationalists and Communists commenced in July 1946. A Chinese general, deciding he wanted the house Sasha was living in for himself, sent fourteen gunmen to seize it. Sasha wasn't sure what to do; she had no legal claim to the house, which Jan had put in Eugenia's name.

So Eugenia made her way to Shanghai to help. There, she found her mother a room and sold as many of their belongings as she could before the general had a chance to appropriate them for himself. While in the city, and despite her earlier attempts to cut things off with him, she resumed her relationship with Avshalomov, who had become conductor of the Shanghai Municipal Council Symphony Orchestra.

When she arrived, Avshalomov was preparing to stage *The Great Wall*, a symphony and ballet based on a tragic folktale about a wife who commits suicide rather than marry the emperor, who has had her husband killed. He hoped to take it on tour throughout Asia before proceeding to the United States. Eugenia had long believed in her lover's talents and wanted to see him thrive. She threw herself into the Chinese Music Drama Association, the group formed to put on the production; in the show's program, she's listed as "Honorary Secretary."

It must have been gratifying to see *The Great Wall* succeed spectacularly. "[T]hose who have seen it are anxious to see it again," raved the *Shanghai Evening Post.* "This is because the show is a great work." That doesn't mean, though, that Eugenia was ready to yoke her life to the composer's.

She still hoped to return to India, but Sasha begged her not to. She feared that her daughter would become a Buddhist nun, lost to the world. Besides, Sasha had heard about the Hindu-Muslim violence that was escalating as India's independence neared. She didn't want to see her daughter caught in yet another civil war. Instead, she and her friends urged Eugenia to go to America. It was, they said, a democratic country, where she'd be free to disseminate her yogic teachings. They talked about the sun in California and the perfume of lemon and orange trees. One of Sasha's friends, Sonia, said that she'd heard about a yoga school opening in Hollywood and suggested that Eugenia would be just the person to lead it. Sonia was going to California herself. They could travel together, and Sonia could make introductions.

Eugenia was torn. She loved India, but she had seen enough war for several lifetimes. Unable to make up her mind, she went to a travel agent and bought two tickets, one for India and the other for the United States. She would leave on whichever ship first departed the Shanghai harbor.

At least, that's the story she would tell later. In fact, she'd received a visa for the United States in New Delhi that August, so she must at least have considered the possibility of a new start in America. Perhaps, as she later nurtured her reputation as the First Lady of Yoga, she felt it difficult to explain why she'd left the country she claimed as her spiritual homeland. If her soul was in India, why was she in Hollywood? It might have felt neater to attribute the move to an accident of chance rather than an act of will. Or maybe she had simply been leaving her options open and had never made up her mind about where her future lay. Either way, she was on the USS *General W. H. Gordon* when it sailed for San Francisco right around New Year's Eve, 1947. Before long, Avshalomov followed her.

· CHAPTER 11 ·

N 1911 the brothers Adolph and Eugene Bernheimer, German-Jewish collectors of Asian art who lived in New York, began work on their summer home in Los Angeles. They dreamed of replicating, in the hills above Hollywood, a palace that was located in the Yamashiro Mountains near Kyoto, and because they were very rich, they brought artisans from Japan to help them. Their teak-and-cedar villa, which took three years to complete, was built around a courtyard and set amid exquisite terraced Japanese gardens with thousands of varieties of trees and plants, not to mention waterfalls, goldfish ponds, and a six-hundred-year-old imported pagoda. The home's circular verandahs offered sweeping views of the Los Angeles Basin, just then being transformed into the capital of American film. The *Los Angeles Times* reported a rumor that the bachelor owners had made a pact that "no woman shall ever enter the place as an invited guest."

It was a pact they couldn't keep. Eugene died in the 1920s, and by the end of the decade their palace had been transformed into the club-house of the Hollywood Four Hundred, an exclusive organization of show business elite. It fell into disrepair during the Depression—rumor has it that it served as a brothel employing desperate actresses. Then came the attack on Pearl Harbor, and the resulting backlash against all things Japanese. Vandals destroyed much of the landscaping, the palace's gorgeous carved wood was painted over, and the estate became a military school. At the war's end, it was transformed once again—into a fifteen-unit apartment building. Thanks to a letter from a friend in Shanghai, that apartment building was where Eugenia settled when she arrived in the United States in 1947.

It was a lucky place to land, close to the action in Hollywood but removed enough to be peaceful, with piney air and lots of tranquil corners conducive to yoga and meditation. Adjusting to a new life in America, Eugenia would depend on both. Contrary to what she'd been told, there was no yoga studio awaiting her. She had no job, no family in the country, and no homeland to return to. She was nearing fifty in a city that worshipped ingénues. She had six thousand dollars in savings—a substantial amount in 1947, but hardly enough to live on. "The only thing left to do," she writes, "was to begin anew."

Still, if she ever panicked, she left no trace of it. Beginning anew was something she was extremely good at, and Los Angeles was the ideal place for it. With World War II, Southern California had become the world capital of the sort of spiritual innovation that flourished in Europe during Eugenia's youth. Krishnamurti had made Ojai, about eighty miles northwest of Los Angeles, his home base. Swami Prabhavananda, a boyish, endlessly patient, chain-smoking monk from Vivekananda's Ramakrishna order, had established a Los Angeles Vedanta Center in 1930. In Hollywood, artists and intellectuals, many of them Europeans driven into exile by the war, flocked to both men. There was a great hunger for the insights of the East adapted to address the malaise of the West.

The fact that Eugenia had so few connections meant she could finally shed her old identity once and for all. Hollywood was a place where people regularly swapped the quotidian names they were born with for more melodious or sophisticated or exotic ones. Many of the people who would become Eugenia's most illustrious students had jettisoned the names their parents gave them—Jennifer Jones was born Phyllis Isley, Ramon Novarro was originally José Ramón

Gil Samaniego, and Greta Garbo had been Greta Gustafsson. In Los Angeles, Eugenia could finally and fully become Indra Devi. Few in America knew her as anything else.

Devi made little effort to contact those who did. Upon arriving, she doesn't seem to have looked up her old master Krishnamurti, which is in some sense surprising—after all, she'd once traveled halfway around the world just to be close to him. A person reinventing herself, though, doesn't always welcome reminders of the past. Krishnamurti knew her as Eugenia, the Theosophist and lovesick diplomatic wife, not as an experienced *yogini*, as women practitioners of yoga are sometimes called. Besides, while Devi was a warm person, she also had a starkly unsentimental side. When a chapter of her life closed, she rarely tried to revisit it, so that people who knew her in one incarnation heard little about those who populated her earlier lives. Leaving the past behind was both a spiritual philosophy and a survival strategy, allowing her to thrive in the midst of calamitous instability. She was generally happy to see people she'd known before, but she didn't seek them out.

In the 1990s, Devi traveled to Moscow to give a talk, accompanied by David and Iana Lifar, the Argentine couple who were her constant companions during the last years of her life. A woman came to her hotel claiming to be the daughter of a cousin of hers, which, if true, would have made her Devi's only known living relative. The two talked for a while, and Devi gave her some money, because she seemed to be quite poor. After forty-five minutes, though, Devi called David and Iana and said that she wanted the woman to go, but she wasn't taking the hint. Iana, who speaks Russian, came and urged her out. The woman was quite upset, telling David and Iana that she hadn't wanted money; she'd wanted to spend time with her "aunt Zhenia."

At breakfast the next morning, David asked Devi why she'd been so eager to get away from the woman. "David," she told him, "I try to live in the eternal now. This lady belongs to my past." She was, for the most part, kind toward those around her, but one of her main teachings, said David, "was not to be attached to anyone," and she practiced it with only a few powerful exceptions.

So, in Los Angeles, rather than seek comfort in her history, Devi steamed forward, looking up Bernardine Fritz, a friend of Emily Hahn's. Fritz had been a doyenne of society in Shanghai, where she'd hosted one of the few salons that brought expatriates together with Chinese artists and intellectuals, though she'd left China before Devi arrived. In Los Angeles, Fritz once again became known as a glittering entertainer, hosting Sunday lunches and cocktail hours in a hilltop home full of Chinese art. She threw a party to introduce Devi to her friends, including many who worked in Hollywood. They gravitated to the exotic newcomer with the saffron sari, eastern European accent, and Indian name.

Fritz was particularly close to Aldous Huxley, who, with his wife, Maria, was at the center of Hollywood's literary and spiritual scenes. As a young British writer, Huxley, a tall and skinny sophisticate who, with his stooped posture and thick glasses, looked rather like a handsome praying mantis, had been famous for his arch skepticism. (One newspaper story about him was headlined "Aldous Huxley: The Man Who Hates God.") Ultimately, though, he found a life of cultivated cynicism insupportable, and under the influence of his friend Gerald Heard, an Anglo-Irish writer who would become one of California's New Age pioneers, he began experimenting with spirituality. (The critic William Tindall lamented Heard's influence on Huxley and mocked their life in California, where, "when they are not walking with Greta Garbo or writing for the cinema, they eat nuts and lettuce perhaps and inoffensively meditate.") Yogic meditation helped Huxley break through a debilitating writer's block. By the time he arrived in the United States for a pacifist lecture tour on the eve of World War II, he was convinced that only spiritual renewal could head off global annihilation.

Though their American sojourn was meant to be temporary, Aldous and Maria ended up settling in Hollywood, where he tried to capitalize on his literary prestige by writing for the movies. They became part of a circle that included Garbo, Charlie Chaplin, Anita Loos, and Christopher Isherwood.

Devi knew Huxley's work, particularly his 1937 book *Ends and Means: An Inquiry into the Nature of Ideals*. She'd quoted it at length in *Yoga: The Technique of Health and Happiness*: "The ideal man is the non-attached man; non-attached to his bodily sensations and lusts; non-attached to his craving for power . . . non-attached to his exclusive loves . . . not even to science, art, speculation, philanthropy."

It's a sign of how quickly Devi moved to the center of things that, soon after arriving in America, she was invited to spend a weekend with the writer and his wife. All that she recorded of this visit is that they discussed health food—Maria warned her that American produce is sprayed with poisonous pesticides.

Like many in Hollywood, the Huxleys experimented with their diets as well as their consciousnesses. "How can you expect to think in anything but a negative way, when you've got chronic intestinal poisoning?" asks the Buddhist Dr. Miller in Huxley's *Eyeless in Gaza*, the 1936 novel that marked the author's turn to the spiritual themes that came to dominate his work. In that book, the narrator, a stand-in for Huxley, moves from jaded libertinism to a desultory stab at guerilla revolution before his encounter with the enlightened doctor saves him. The doctor lectures him on "the correlation between religion and diet . . . The fact is, of course, that we think as we eat."

Everywhere in the emerging New Age culture was an assumed connection between health and salvation. That link, of course, is at the heart of modern hatha yoga's power. (It exists in evangelical Christianity, too, but the cause and effect are reversed: salvation can lead to health, rather than vice versa.) Yoga as it eventually came to be practiced in the United States elevates exercise into a sacrament, merging the contradictory quests for beauty and selflessness. It's a kind of secular magic, promising that by assuming certain physical positions, you can bring about specific changes in the body and

soul—clearer skin and clearer thoughts. It's alchemy for a disenchanted age, rendered plausible to Westerners by translating esoteric
tantric terms into the language of glands and hormones. Yet, until
Devi arrived, no one in Los Angeles was teaching it.

There had been hatha yoga teachers in the United States before,
most famously Pierre Bernard, né Perry Baker, who, as an occult-
minded teenager in 1889, had the fantastic good luck to meet a
tantric yogi in Lincoln, Nebraska. Sylvais Hamati, who had come
from Calcutta, may have worked on the western railroads or, as Robert Love, Bernard's biographer writes, he may have been a traveling entertainer, "a mind reader or a hypnotist, like 'Professor Craig
of Hebron, the boy prodigy' who promised Nebraskans he could
place a subject in a 'cataleptic state' for five days." Hamati taught
Bernard "advanced physical culture" (i.e., asanas), *pranayama*, and
meditation.

Bernard first used his skills as a sideshow performer in San Francisco, putting himself into a trance and lying tranquil while his
assistant inserted a needle through his lip and cheek and a hatpin
through his tongue. He started a secret society known as the Tantrik
Order, "a band of dashing gypsy occultists who traveled in a pack,
lived together in communes, and conducted their mystical business
late in the evenings," as Love writes, business that included various
sexual rites.

In 1910, Bernard was the subject of major national scandal in
New York, charged with abducting two of his young female pupils,
both of whom he was sleeping with. "'Hindoo Priest' Lures Girls . . .
Weird Dance His Cure," blared the *Chicago Daily Tribune*. "Wild
Orgies in the Temple of 'Om,'" screamed the *San Francisco Chronicle*. He was held for three months in New York's infamous Tombs
before the case fell apart; though the charges were ultimately dismissed, he was disgraced.

Bernard's arrest was just one of several American yoga scandals
that took place in the early twentieth century. "Coroner Holds
'Hindu Yogi,'" read a 1910 *New York Tribune* headline about the

arrest of Samri Ellis—his real name was Charles F. Balwanz—in the shooting death of his assistant. The same year, the *Los Angeles Times* reported on the arrest of Sakharam G. Pandit, "the Hindu with the 'hypnotic eye,' whose Oriental religious practices have been denounced by many of his women students." In 1911 the paper ran a story about women who had "abandoned home and husband and children to join the sun worshippers in the study of yoga." Its headline: "A Hindu Apple for Modern Eve: The Cult of the Yogis Lures Women to Destruction."

Unlike most other tabloid yogis, Bernard was able to rebuild his reputation, attracting socialites and celebrities such as cosmetics queen Helena Rubinstein, actress Ethel Barrymore, and Frances Payne Bolton, later the first woman elected to Congress from Ohio. Eventually, he founded the Clarkstown Country Club in Nyack, New York, a Jazz Age destination where a fashionable crowd enjoyed asana classes, concerts, baseball games, and elaborate amateur circuses. "Lawyers and teachers and heiresses would be transformed into clowns, tumblers, high-wire artists, magicians, trapezists, animal trainers, barkers and prop masters," writes Love.

The Clarkstown Country Club wasn't the only place teaching hatha yoga in upstate New York in the early 1920s. After founding the Yoga Institute in a suburb of Bombay in 1918, Sri Yogendra came to the United States, hoping to popularize his hatha system. In 1920 he set up a yoga institute on Bear Mountain in Harriman, New York, working with medical doctors and meeting American health gurus such as Bernarr Macfadden and John Harvey Kellogg.

But Yogendra stayed in the country less than five years, and thanks to the Immigration Act of 1924, which banned East Asians and Indians from coming to live in the United States, he was unable to return. The Clarkstown Country Club fell into disrepair during the Depression, and yoga retained its reputation as something racy, disreputable, and perhaps a bit ridiculous. Edith Wharton's satirical 1927 novel *Twilight Sleep* features a society matron in thrall to a "Mahatma" whose "eurythmic exercises . . . had reduced her hips after everything else had failed." She later works furiously to quash an incipient scandal involving several young socialites, her daughter-in-law among them, implicated in lascivious activities at the mahatma's retreat center, "Dawnside."

When Devi arrived in Los Angeles, there were one or two people in California who'd been trained by Bernard and offered private lessons, but the field was largely empty. Indeed, when Devi gave a lecture to celebrity nutritionist Gayelord Hauser's "Eaters Anonymous" group in Los Angeles, one attendee listened to the whole thing thinking that it was about yogurt.

Yet if most Los Angelinos didn't know what hatha yoga was, many were eager to learn, given the growing fashion for Eastern spirituality and the perennial obsession with improving the body. Encouraged by Fritz and her friends, Devi leased a studio at 8806 Sunset Boulevard, on the notorious Sunset Strip. (The legendary nightclubs Mocambo and Ciro's were both a few blocks away.) Her classes were only moderately challenging and resolutely free of religion; she went to great pains to explain the practice in scientific rather than spiritual terms. Yoga, as she presented it, was first and foremost a commonsense exercise and relaxation system, utterly practical and wholesome, promising transformative results without the grunting agony of other physical culture regimens.

Slowly, her fame started building, initially under the name Indira Devi, which she still sometimes used during her first couple of years in Hollywood. In February 1949, Paul Bragg, former wrestler, bodybuilder, and nationally famous health food guru, hosted a three-night lecture series for her at LA's fifteen-hundred-seat Embassy Auditorium. "Her amazing exhibition of Yoga Health exercises will leave you breathless!" promised an ad in the *Los Angeles Times*. "Indira Devi shows how to recharge the batteries of your mind and body with Vital Cosmic Energy."

Devi's mother soon followed her to the United States, which surely pleased her. Soon Sasha was creating a life of her own in California—shortly after she arrived, she married George Ghermanoff, a Turkish-born actor who was a couple of years younger than she. (He'd had tiny, uncredited roles in Cecil B. DeMille's *The Buccaneer* and Rouben Mamoulian's *The Mark of Zorro*.) It's not clear if she was still living with Devi in the summer of 1948, when Avshalomov arrived, uninvited, and moved into Devi's apartment in the Yamashiro building.

Unlike Devi, Avshalomov had a hard time gaining a foothold in Los Angeles. He hoped to stage *The Great Wall* there and to make money by writing scores for movies. While Devi tried to use her growing connections on his behalf, none of his plans came to anything. Broke, he considered taking a job in a record shop, but was ultimately too proud. He was not, however, too proud to let Devi support him; even after he found his own apartment, she paid his rent. This could not have been easy for her, since money was tight. To raise funds, she managed, through an intermediary, to sell what remained of her and Strakaty's interest in the Shanghai noodle company, for which she received $4,500.

Struggling, Avshalomov talked about going back to Shanghai. "[P]robably when I am finally convinced that all my efforts here are in vain, I will take that step—much as I would hate to lose face," he writes. His inability to take care of himself maddened his son, who had a budding music career of his own. "I felt that underlying his inability to get professional work as a musician was his 19th century assumption that society owed it to artists to support them," writes Jacob. It must have frustrated Devi as well, though she never wrote a word about it—a depressed, deadbeat, married Russian boyfriend wouldn't have been helpful to the image she was cultivating.

Avshalomov hoped to bring his wife, Tanya, to the United States and imagined that he could remain married to her while continuing his affair with Devi. "No matter what I do I will hurt some one badly," he writes. "I cant [*sic*] be cruel to Tanya and leave her, my only hope is that she will agree to tolerate a triangular situation. Asking too much, I know. Yet my feelings toward both women are deep and sincere."

Meanwhile, though Devi didn't know it, this love triangle was threatening her future in the United States. Around the time that Avshalomov left China for California, someone sent an anonymous letter to the American consulate in Shanghai accusing Devi of being an "important Soviet agent." The author had an imperfect command of English, writing, "Before this war she spent few years in India, where she learned Ioga's [*sic*] science and exercises and married old and rich Czech commercial ahache [*sic*]." Though Devi is "not yong" [*sic*] and "not pretty," the writer said, she is "very intelligent" and has "very attractive manners." Under the "veil" of yoga, the letter said, she had "penetrated everywhere."

The charge was absurd, as everyone whom the FBI interviewed about Devi pointed out. Edwin Stanton, the former American consul in Shanghai and husband of one of her first students, Josie, vouched for her, writing that although the "philosophical concepts of yoga . . . are very broad and liberal in nature, neither I nor my wife recollect ever hearing her make any statements or remarks which would indicate that she is a Communist or 'a fellow traveler.'" Colonel M. B. DePass, who had been an American military attaché in Shanghai, told the FBI that he believed Devi would make a good American citizen. Less kindly, the American judge Milton Helmick told investigators that Devi couldn't possibly be a Soviet agent because she wasn't "sufficiently intelligent or discreet to be entrusted by the Soviets with undercover assignments." DePass's former secretary, another of Devi's students, told investigators that the anonymous letter must have come from Tanya Avshalomov. When Devi was finally interviewed, she had the same suspicion.

Yet proving her innocence wasn't easy. This was the height of the McCarthy era. Congressional hearings into Communist subversion in Hollywood had been going on since 1947. Devi was a Russian with multiple aliases and a suspiciously bohemian lifestyle. When FBI agents first reported that they had found nothing incriminating about Indra Devi, Hoover told them to look harder. "In view of the original allegations in this case it is not believed that sufficient investigation has been conducted to definitely disprove those allegations," he writes in a March 16, 1950, memo about her.

This was a problem for Devi. Her status in the country was tenuous. With the Communist takeover of Czechoslovakia, Jan's diplomatic career had come to an end, and the new regime refused to let him leave the country. Devi had entered the United States as the wife of a diplomat; when the Immigration and Naturalization Service realized that her husband had no official status, she was told she couldn't stay. Being under investigation as a Communist agent didn't help her case. One June 13, 1950, with her status still unresolved, a warrant was issued for her arrest.

VEN AS her immigration struggles threatened to derail her American life, Devi was thriving as never before, as socialites and actresses began to discover what yoga could do for them. In 1950 she was invited to teach at an outpost of Elizabeth Arden's Maine Chance spa near Phoenix, Arizona, where for around four hundred dollars a week—more than thirty-eight hundred in today's dollars—wealthy women went to live in "sumptuous starvation," in the words of *Life* magazine. Days passed in a tightly regimented schedule of exercise classes and beauty treatments. It was as square an environment as could be imagined, a place where spiritual aspiration, if it existed, was sublimated into a Sisyphean battle against weight gain and aging. Devi was extremely well received, and by teaching there, she both popularized and further domesticated yoga, turning it into a hobby for respectable bourgeois ladies. This is one of the ironies of hatha yoga in America: rich housewives discovered it well before it became the avant-garde enthusiasm of beats and hippies.

Arden, the perpetually pink-clad creator of a cosmetics empire, was a Canadian parvenu with a weakness for aristocrats. She had a special fondness for White Russians and a long-standing fascination with yoga. She must have been happy to find Devi, an expert asana teacher with excellent social credentials and no hint of the sort of impropriety associated with earlier generations of American yogis. After a stint in Arizona, Devi, ignoring the warrant for her arrest, spent the summer season at Arden's original Maine Chance spa, in Mount Vernon, Maine. In the fall, Arden brought Devi to New York City to instruct her personally.

There, Devi ran into an old friend whom she hadn't seen in more than thirty years: Valentina Sanina. The last time they'd been together, in Kharkov after the Russian Revolution, Valentina had been an icy, remote ingénue pursued by Alexander Vertinsky. She'd come to New York in 1923 with her husband, George Schlee, and had become one of the country's most celebrated fashion designers, known for her rigorously spare, architectural, wildly expensive couture. Valentina—she was by then known by only one name—dressed the most ravishing figures in Hollywood, many of whom would later become Devi's students. No one was closer to her, though, than Greta Garbo.

During the 1940s, Valentina, Schlee, and Garbo formed an inseparable triad. The exact romantic dynamic between them all is hard to discern. At the time, the rumor was that Valentina was sharing her husband with the actress, though it's also possible that Valentina and Garbo, who had at least one female ex-lover in common, were romantically involved as well. Whatever her relationship with the Schlees, when she was with them, the usually retiring Garbo courted gossip: "The two women would dress in identical Valentina ensembles for high-profile nights out on the town—with George in the middle, Garbo on one arm, and Valentina on the other," writes Valentina's biographer. Here was an acquaintanceship Devi was happy to renew.

When Devi showed up in New York, the threesome was fraying, with Garbo and Schlee settling into coupledom, to Valentina's dismay.* Still, Valentina was at least outwardly friendly with Garbo,

---

*Garbo eventually bought an apartment in the same building as the one Schlee and his wife shared on East Fifty-Second Street, and Valentina came to hate the

and she introduced Devi to the legendary actress. Garbo already knew something of yoga—in the 1930s she'd had an affair with the conductor Leopold Stokowski, a health fanatic who'd frequented Pierre Bernard's Clarkstown Country Club. Thanks to Avshalomov, Devi knew Stokowski as well. The two women also had other friends, including the Huxleys, in common. Garbo was happy to hear that Devi had opened a studio in Los Angeles, and promised to come when she was on the West Coast.

She did, and other stars did, too. Jennifer Jones took classes; a cameraman on her movie *Gone to Earth* complained about her habit of "standing on her head for several minutes just before a take while the assembled company waited in expectation." Marion Mill Preminger, then the bored, frustrated wife of the director Otto Preminger, went, but struggled with the meditation at the end of class. "During one yoga lesson I was feeling very discouraged, thinking I should have gone to the jiujitsu [*sic*] lesson instead," she recalled. "Just then I heard Indra saying, 'Everybody look at Marion in the Lotus Position. She sits like a flower. She looks like a flower. She even thinks like a flower.'"

Robert Balzer, the country's preeminent wine writer and a prominent man-about-town, noticed that several friends "had taken on a new radiant vitality" after practicing with Devi. He began working with her as well, both at her Sunset Boulevard studio and on the lawn of his hilltop home in Beverly Hills, and soon he introduced her to his lover, Gloria Swanson. At the time, Swanson was enjoying a sort of Hollywood comeback, having just played the monstrous Norma Desmond, decayed relic of the silent film era, in *Sunset Bou-*

---

actress. After George Schlee's death, the two women remained locked in a sort of cold war, each refusing to move but doing everything possible to avoid each other, though in a 1978 letter to Devi written in rhyming doggerel (and signed, jokingly, Maharajah Indor Schlee), Valentina seems less hostile than gently mocking: "I hope that my friend 'that wants to be alone' / Exercises in the open air, on her own lawn / As I think it will do her a lot of good / And keep her always in an excelent [*sic*] mood."

levard, Billy Wilder's Grand Guignol masterpiece about the horror of aging in Hollywood.

As a silent film star, Swanson had been the highest-paid actress of her day, and many people thought that Norma Desmond was an exaggerated version of her. The film made use of old Swanson footage; a clip meant to show Norma in her glory days came from *Queen Kelly*, a failed 1929 movie produced by Swanson's ex-lover Joe Kennedy. After *Sunset Boulevard* came out, Swanson wrote of being bombarded with scripts "that were awful imitations of Sunset Boulevard, all featuring a deranged superstar crashing toward tragedy."

Yet Swanson, who was born the same year as Devi, was no Norma Desmond, and handled aging much better than many in her cohort, finding other pursuits when her career went into decline. In the late 1930s she'd formed a company, Multiprises, which brought to the United States scientists escaping Hitler's Germany and financed their inventions in return for a share of the profits. Before *Sunset Boulevard*, she'd hosted one of the first live television talk shows, *The Gloria Swanson Hour*. Afterward, she acted on Broadway and started a fashion design business, helming a line called "Forever Young." Long a vegetarian and, in her own words, a "fanatic about healthy food," she campaigned against agricultural pesticides. (In 1976 she wed her sixth husband, William Dufty, the author of the health food tome *Sugar Blues*, which is still influential today.) An enthusiastic yoga student, Swanson became Devi's closet friend in Hollywood, propelling Devi's career and, with it, yoga's popularity.

The FBI kept following Devi, though no attempts were made to deport her. Meanwhile, as her renown grew, the publisher Prentice Hall contracted her to write a book. Sidney Field, a screenwriter who was the son of leading Theosophists, helped with the manuscript. Swanson suggested the title, based on the name of her fashion line, and *Forever Young, Forever Healthy* was published in the fall of 1953. The actress provided a cover endorsement, and other blurbs came from Linda Christian, soon to become the first Bond girl, and from the modern dance pioneer Ruth St. Denis, Martha Graham's teacher.

Forever Young, Forever Healthy is largely antimystical, as much an all-purpose self-help tome as a yoga treatise. Devi promises to teach readers how to sleep better, feel calmer and more cheerful, lose or gain weight, even rid themselves of wrinkles. The book combines lessons she learned from Krishnamacharya and Kuvalayananda with elements of New Thought and nature cure and even a light sprinkling of feminism. Its tone alternates between sternness and affectionate exasperation. "I shall not even make an attempt to persuade heavy smokers to give up their cigarettes or cigars, as they are not going to do it anyway," she writes, proposing that smokers instead practice deep breathing to mitigate the effects of their habit.

A chapter on diet includes commonsense instructions to avoid fried foods and refined sugar, and recommends vegetable juice and soy. It instructs readers to ignore stories they've heard "about someone's 'uncle' who ate everything, drank everything, did everything wrong and yet lived to be a hundred." You, she writes, "are not this superman uncle, or you wouldn't be reading this book."

Toward the end of the book is a chapter titled "The Woman Beautiful," which encapsulates Devi's combination of pitilessness and encouragement. It begins with Devi urging women to stand naked before a full-length mirror and conduct frank self-appraisals, her words reading like the dictates of a cruel sorority sister. Ask yourself, she urges, what you don't like about your body. "Your hips perhaps? Or your stomach?" Then, she continues, figure out what you did to make it that way. Is it because you take too many drinks, or eat too much or smoke too much . . . Or perhaps you are too lazy and do not exercise enough." Not for Devi the gospel of self-acceptance. Her message was clear: if you're not beautiful, it's your fault.

Yet, in a style later perfected by countless women's magazines, she follows up her undermining with a message of empowerment, telling women to attend to their looks in order to be confident of their femininity as they move out of traditional roles. Women, she writes, are moving through a period of historical transformation: "Being awakened to a new freedom, they will probably have to suffer even more now than they did a generation ago when they lacked it."

Ultimately, she believed, the growing antagonism between the sexes "will continue until man grants woman equality as a human being," but she urges women to maintain their femininity even as they compete with men economically. "She must stop imitating him, his attitude and manners, and become intrinsically herself," she writes.

By today's standards, this seems a bit reactionary. But in 1953, with much of the country in thrall to the stifling cult of domesticity that Betty Friedan describes in *The Feminine Mystique*, parts of Devi's message would have seemed liberating. Other self-help books of the time acknowledged that women were restless and unhappy, and blamed it on their failure to adapt to a life of housewifery. The enormously influential, viciously antifeminist book *Modern Woman: The Lost Sex* published in 1947, claims that women were suffering because they'd attempted to find satisfaction "by the route of male achievement" instead of the female path of nurture. Devi, by contrast, assumed women were suffering because they wanted equality but didn't yet have it, and she offered a soothing ritual to help them cope in the meantime.

Pop Freudianism was increasingly influential in the 1950s and was frequently used to castigate women for what one writer called a "masculinity complex." (One of the coauthors of *Modern Woman: The Lost Sex* was the psychoanalyst Marynia Farnham.) In her book, Devi borrows from Freud as well, but to different ends. "It is a well known fact that sex repression often results in sadism, masochism, extreme cruelty and other abnormalities," she writes. She is firm about the duty of men to please their wives sexually and says little about the reverse. Sex, she writes, is a "very important, if not all-important, factor in marriage and an emotionally mature and loving husband is the best person to help his wife to overcome her frigidity, provided he himself hasn't caused it by being a clumsy, crude, and uninspiring lover."

None of this has much to do with yoga, but it certainly spoke to the frustrations that, at the time of the book's publication, drove at least some people to the practice. And though traditionally yoga had been employed to sublimate the libido, Devi writes that for Westerners, it could help people express their sexual energies "more beautifully and more fully than they ever have before."

Only in the last forty pages does Devi get into asanas, giving instructions for familiar poses such as the plow, bow, lotus, shoulder stand, and headstand. Initially, she and Swanson did a photo shoot to accompany this section, practicing together outdoors in front of a flowering hedge. In one picture, they stand side by side with opposite legs in half lotus, their knees touching. They're the same height, and both all in black; Swanson is wearing a strapless tank top with a jaunty little bow around her neck.

At the last minute, though, Swanson informed Devi that Prentice Hall had decided to save the pictures for the book *she* was writing, the never-completed *Beauty after Forty*. There was little Devi could say; Swanson was by far the more famous and powerful of the pair. Instead, Devi appears in the book's photos either alone or guiding a group of a half-dozen female students, most with full makeup and pin-curled hair, looking almost like chorus girls. Jack Macfadden, stepson of the exercise guru Bernarr Macfadden, posed for a few shots as well, including one of the difficult peacock pose, an arm balance in which the rest of the body is held off the ground horizontally, parallel to the floor.

Swanson helped launch the book, presenting Devi and *Forever Young, Forever Healthy* to a crowd of fashionable women and curious journalists at New York's Waldorf-Astoria hotel. Walter Winchell, the gimlet-eyed gossip writer, mentioned the event in his syndicated column, which appeared in more than two thousand newspapers: "Gloria Swanson's latest 'kick'—introducing her Yoga to socialites."

Forever Young, Forever Healthy quickly became a best seller, spreading Devi's fame nationwide. "Among the 'sideline' stars of Hollywood is Indra Devi, who teaches movie stars to eat moss and potato water, stand on their heads, cut down on romance and tie their legs into knots," began a wire service story on Devi. The "discomfort . . . known as yoga," continued reporter Aline Mosby, "appeals to such luminaries as Robert Ryan, Suzanne Ball, Gloria Swanson, Linda Christian and Jennifer Jones." Visiting Devi's studio, "one of the curiosities of the Sunset Strip," Mosby didn't see the appeal. The class, she wrote, consisted of "Indra standing on her head and me trying a leg-knotting torture known as the 'lotus position.'"

Other journalists proved gamer. Jack Zaiman, a columnist for the *Hartford Courant*, described trying to do a headstand at the YMCA after reading the book. "What are you doing?" asked his friend Wardy Waterman. "I'm a Yoga," Zaiman replied proudly, before crashing to the floor.

Soon Prentice Hall signed Devi up for two more books. She criss-crossed the country giving lectures, often trying, at the request of her many hosts, to rope Swanson into appearing with her. PLEASE DO NOT INVOLVE ME IN ANY SPEECHES, LUNCHEONS OR ANYTHING ELSE, Swanson cabled Devi on February 15, 1954. I WILL ONLY HAVE A FEW DAYS WHICH I HOPE TO SPEND WITH MY FAMILY AND FEW FRIENDS BEFORE I START A VERY STRENUOUS TOUR. WOULD YOU PLEASE SEND ME THE NAME OF XXXXX THE DOCTOR WHO WROTE A BOOK ON FEET. LOVE GLORIA.

If there was a note of rebuke in Swanson's message, Devi doesn't seem to have picked up on it. Perhaps she was too happy to register anything negative. At fifty-four, she had finally found major profes-sional success. Perhaps more important, she was in love again, and not with Avshalomov. Further, thanks to her new partner, all her immigration problems were about to disappear. At the end of a four-page letter to Swanson—Devi addressed her as "my beloved"—she gushed over her renewed sense of tranquility and joy by the side of a "saint in disguise." Her words made it clear that this saint was someone Swanson knew well. Both she and her paramour, wrote Devi, "think about you, talk about you, and love you, my wonderful Gloria."

SASHA'S MARRIAGE to Ghermanoff didn't last, and by the 1950s, she was once again living with Devi. Sometime in 1951 or 1952 she grew sick. In her autobiography, Devi says that Sasha developed a heart condition, but in reality, she had breast cancer, a disease that was then wrapped up with stigma and shame. It was natural that Devi would take her to see Sigfrid Knauer, a German doctor living in Los Angeles. He was known for his spiritualism and for alternative cancer treatments such as Iscador, derived from mistletoe, a remedy that today is widely used in some European countries but considered quackery by most mainstream American doctors.

While in Knauer's office, Devi said something private to her mother in Russian, assuming the doctor wouldn't understand. When he spoke to her in Russian in response, she blushed. They started talking, and she learned that they'd traveled similar trajectories in their early lives. She quickly came to feel a deep connection with him.

Born in Kiev in 1894, Sigfrid Knauer studied medicine at Germany's University of Jena before becoming a pupil of the Austrian mystic Rudolf Steiner, a onetime leader of the Theosophical Society in Germany, Switzerland, and the Austro-Hungarian Empire.

Unlike most prominent Theosophists, Steiner rooted his spirituality in the esoteric Christian tradition, not Eastern religion. (He did, however, incorporate ideas of karma and rebirth.) As Theosophy became increasingly identified with Hinduism and Buddhism, Steiner moved away from it, finally splitting with the society over Annie Besant's deification of Krishnamurti. In 1913 he founded his own movement, the Anthroposophical Society.

Under its banner, Steiner undertook an epic number of projects. He developed all-encompassing theories of political and social organization meant to rival capitalism and communism. He elaborated a metaphysical doctrine in which humankind is menaced by two sinister forces—Lucifer, the spirit of pride, and Ahriman, the spirit of materialism. He had theories about art and architecture that he put into practice in building his grand headquarters in Switzerland, the Goetheanum, after Johann Wolfgang von Goethe.

His pedagogical system has had the most far-reaching impact; Waldorf schools, with their emphasis on nurturing the creativity and uniqueness of every student, have been very influential in the world of progressive private education. But for Indra Devi's story, what's most important is Steiner's creation, in concert with Ita Wegman, of Anthroposophical medicine.

Like many practitioners of homeopathic medicine, Steiner believed that illness stems from imbalances in the body, but in his view, the body can't be limited to material, physical processes. "Man is what he is through physical body, ether body, soul (astral body) and I (spirit)," Steiner and Wegman write in their book *Extending Practical Medicine: Fundamental Principles Based on the Science of the Spirit.* Illness, they argue, is an upset in the balance between these elements, and for health, "it is necessary to find medicines that will restore the upset balance." (The etheric body, in this formulation, might be analogized to the concept of energy, or *prana*, in yogic thought.)

Using these principles, Steiner developed an entire pharmacopeia. Anthroposophic medicine is often based on concordances between physical substances and bodily dysfunctions, in which like is thought to cure like. So, for example, rock salt is used to treat diseases including chronic rhinitis (stuffy, runny nose) because salt, like mucus, can be both crusty and, when dissolved, liquid. Anthroposophic medicine is intended to complement, rather than replace, Western medicine. Doctors working in the field are supposed to get conventional medical degrees and then supplement their knowledge with Steiner's system for gaining spiritual and even supernatural insights—which is precisely what Knauer had done.

Knauer had an Anthroposophical medical practice in pre–World War II Berlin, where he served as the doctor at the local Waldorf School and, according to an obituary, treated various aristocrats. When the Nazis came to power, he, his wife, Edith, and their four children fled the country, landing in New York in 1939. Unable to get a medical license in that state, he set out for Los Angeles, where he became the doctor to the local Anthroposophical community and to artists, celebrities, and ordinary people who turned to alternative medicine when conventional cures failed them.

Like his mentor, Knauer rejected a materialistic explanation of ill health. "Illness is a part of man's evolution," he writes. "It is a challenge, a warning, a stimulation. It is an indication that man has failed somewhere. To overcome this . . . [h]e has to realize that he stands with his ego between the spiritual and the earthly worlds and that he has to strengthen his spiritual forces to be able to integrate them into his earthly existence."

Yet Knauer didn't practice mind cure; he incorporated all sorts of physical techniques and substances into his work. He took what he learned from Steiner and built on it, drawing on acupuncture and Russian folk medicine—and, later, yoga. Often, he used a pendulum to make diagnoses. "He would have a shelf full of little medicines, just crowded with little bottles," one of his patients, John Brousseau, told me. "He didn't advertise it much, but he would have a little silver pendulum in one hand, and he would pick up the particular medicine and place it on the spot that was giving trouble. And depending on the pendulum, it would either go back and forth or it would go round and round in a circle." The motion, says Brousseau, would tell Knauer whether or not his patient had a "harmonic convergence with the substance."

Eccentric as this may sound, Knauer's patients considered him an unparalleled healer. Some still talk about his bedside manner—the warmth behind his brusque, dry sense of humor. "He was a very sharp wit, but he was very gentle," says Jean Brousseau, John's wife. "His hands were so gentle."

In her memoir, Devi says that Knauer cured her mother, but in fact she needed a mastectomy. Nevertheless, her faith in his healing powers was strong, and shortly after they met, when she needed medical advice for a chapter in *Forever Young, Forever Healthy*, she turned to her new friend, and eventually a romance developed.

Knauer had lost his first wife to cancer in 1948, a death that haunted him and spurred his obsession with the disease. When Devi met him, he was married to his second wife, the gorgeous, blonde, and much younger Vera von Hossenfeldt von Langer Wisbar, the daughter of a German insurance salesman. Described by one writer as "one of history's most infamous and unabashed gold-diggers," Vera had become a baroness thanks to her first husband. An aspiring actress, she then traded the baron for the director Frank Wisbar, and together they left Germany for Los Angeles after the start of World War II. But Wisbar failed to make inroads at any of the American studios, and Vera was reduced to working as a department store salesgirl and then as Knauer's receptionist. Evidently, Knauer seemed a better prospect than the husband she had, so she secured a divorce from Wisbar in Las Vegas and married her boss.

The union was short-lived. A few months after Devi met Knauer, Vera left him and decamped to Germany, where, in 1952, she married Alfried Krupp, the German industrialist and Nazi war criminal. A major supplier of weaponry to Hitler's regime and an enthusiastic employer of slave labor, Krupp had been sentenced by the Allies to twelve years in prison for crimes against humanity. Vera, who had known Krupp in her youth, wrote to him when he was locked up. When, after three years, the U.S. High Commissioner for Germany arranged to have him pardoned, she and Krupp fell into each other's arms. As a wedding gift, Krupp gave his new bride the most expensive Porsche on the market.

It seems fair to assume that Knauer was eager to move on. In Devi he found a partner, a woman who spoke his languages and shared his background and his passions. He adored her catalyzing energy. Later in life, he would often tell friends that she was an "activator—wherever she goes, she awakens and quickens and activates things." They were married on March 14, 1953, and bought a house in Hollywood with a secluded open patio facing Nichols Canyon. Devi insisted on separate bedrooms, believing that privacy and autonomy were both spiritually necessary and key to lasting romance. Her indulgent, gallant new husband—whom she always called "Doctor"—ended her immigration problems, since he was an American citizen. There's no record of her divorcing Strakaty, though if she was a bigamist, no authority noticed.

Avshalomov was blindsided, telling his son that he'd been left for a hypnotist. Tanya felt vindicated, writing to Avshalomov's son, "I begged him to leave her, predicted what would happen. But he said he would never leave her, would rather leave me. So he did, and I dont [*sic*] want him back."

<hr>

Together, Devi and Knauer formed an alternative-medicine power couple. While Devi instructed movie stars, Knauer became the private physician to the celebrated composer Igor Stravinsky, a close friend of Aldous Huxley. "Knauer, together with his Russian-born and Indian bred wife, Indra Devi, deserves a place in any biography of Stravinsky in the Hollywood years; by age, cultural background . . . and holistic medical philosophy, he was closer to Stravinsky than any of his other American-period physicians," writes the composer's friend and biographer Robert Craft.

Some who loved Stravinsky thought Knauer a dangerous crank. A book that Stravinsky's second wife, Vera, cowrote with Craft laments the way the composer fell under the influence of his idiosyncratic doctor, with his "homeopathic prescriptions, his system of diagnoses by pendulum, and his belief in rejuvenation by the ingestion of minced fetuses."

There's no evidence that this last, ghoulish detail was true, but some of Knauer's remedies were unusual even by the standards of alternative medicine. Brenda Barnetson, Jean Brousseau's sister, recalls Knauer giving shots of a preparation he said was made with ground dinosaur fossils, a treatment for radiation poisoning, which he believed was endemic. "When you got an injection of this, your body went *whoosh* and warmed up; it was amazing," she says.

However strange his methods, he evoked intense loyalty among many patients. His practice was so full that even the very famous would wait hours for appointments at his Sunset Boulevard office. "His other patients often proved fascinating as they all waited together, such as Marilyn Monroe, Dale Evans, Michael Chekhov . . . and others," writes Henry Barnes, a historian of the Steiner movement. "Igor Stravinsky would keep Mala Powers fascinated in the waiting room as he read musical scores the way most people read books."

Devi's career was thriving as well. Interest in yoga was growing all over the country, in part because of mounting concern about the toll that stress was taking on Americans' health. Stress is now such a ubiquitous concept that it's hard to imagine that it hasn't always been with us, but according to Anne Harrington, a historian of science at Harvard, preoccupation with stress didn't become widespread until the 1950s. That's when Hans Selye, a physician and biochemist at the University of Montreal, formulated the idea that a constant state of tension or alarm creates a cascading hormonal reaction that, if unrelieved, causes chronic, predictable physical damage. He called this state "stress," a term he took from metallurgy. It quickly came to replace the earlier concept of neurasthenia, which was seen as a nervous disorder brought about by chronic exhaustion and was treated, at least in women, with total bed rest and a heavy diet.

Selye's scientific colleagues were skeptical at first, but the general public embraced the idea, happy to have a name for the inchoate but widely shared feeling of anxious malaise brought on by modern life. The 1950s, after all, was a worry-choked decade. The threat of nuclear annihilation thrummed relentlessly in the background even as the country reveled in a Technicolor consumerist boom. Fleeing the cities for exploding suburbs, young families found themselves cut off from traditional social networks. The cult of domesticity kept many women isolated in their homes and feeling ashamed of their lack of fulfillment there. Men, toiling in increasingly impersonal bureaucracies, experienced another sort of relentless pressure; as Harrington points out, these were the years that gave us expressions such as the "rat race."

Popular books of the time worried about this constant low-level unease. David Riesman's epochal *The Lonely Crowd* diagnosed a new middle class made up of "other-directed" people, conformists who constantly recalibrated their ideas about how to live based on the lives of their peers. Writes Riesman, "The other-directed person must be able to receive signals from far and near; the sources are many, the changes rapid . . . [O]ne prime psychological lever of the other-directed person is a diffuse *anxiety*" (his italics).

Beneath their surface placidity, Americans were desperate for relief. When the pharmaceutical company Carter-Wallace introduced Miltown, the first prescription minor tranquilizer, in 1955, it quickly because the fastest-selling drug in U.S. history. (By 1957, an astonishing third of all prescriptions were for tranquilizers.) The pills were particularly popular in Hollywood, where the famous Schwab's drugstore on Sunset Boulevard couldn't keep them in stock. A 1955 ad in the *Los Angeles Times* trumpeted: "Attention physicians: just arrived by air, another shipment of MILTOWN. Your prescriptions can now be filled.

For those who wanted a different kind of balm, yoga beckoned. "Before a new student joins my class, he is usually asked, among other things, what is his reason for taking up Yoga," writes Devi. "The great majority, I find, want to learn how to relax . . . One constantly hears people saying, 'I am all on edge,' 'My nerves are in bad shape,' 'It's nothing but my poor nerves.'"

As it happens, yoga is uniquely suited to addressing stress. Researchers have found that some of the most common Western claims for the benefits of yoga, particularly the type of gentle hatha yoga Devi taught, are overblown. Many people take up yoga to lose weight, but it turns out that the practice can actually lower the metabolism rather than raise it, meaning that, in the words of one physiologist, it can create "a propensity for weight gain and fat deposition." Even the most vigorous styles of yoga do little for aerobic conditioning. A 2010 review of more than eighty studies of yoga and other types of exercise found that yoga improved people's lives as much or more than conventional workouts in a whole host of ways—save "those involving physical fitness," a rather significant exception.

Yet if yoga doesn't generally burn calories, it does wonders for the nervous system. The 2010 review found that yoga decreases blood pressure, "reverses the negative impact of stress on the immune system," lowers anxiety, and increases "feelings of emotional, social, and spiritual well-being." Further, it is more beneficial than other types of exercise in reducing fatigue and sleep disturbance. The review speculated that yoga works by calming the sympathetic nervous system and what's called the hypothalamic-pituitary-adrenal axis, which produces stress hormones. Yoga, it seems, can actually help undo the body's natural but maladaptive response to the modern world. No wonder the more overwhelming the postwar world seemed, the more people flocked to it.

Among those who did was Yehudi Menuhin, one of the greatest violinists of the twentieth century. A child prodigy who performed his first violin solo with the San Francisco Symphony Orchestra at the age of seven, Menuhin fell into an artistic funk after World War II. He discovered yoga when he picked up a book about it in the waiting room of a New Zealand osteopath and taught himself some asanas. In 1952, while on tour in India, he boasted to local newspapers about his ability to stand on his head, prompting Jawaharlal Nehru to goad him into a demonstration, in full evening dress, during a state banquet. The prime minister informed him that he had a long way to go and proceeded to demonstrate proper form as assorted dignitaries looked on. Later, India's president arranged for Menuhin to attend a class taught by the country's oldest practicing yogi. Then, in Bombay, the violinist began searching for a teacher who could travel with him.

He was, according to his biographer, besieged by offers. The person he finally chose was Krishnamacharya's brother-in-law B. K. S. Iyengar. When Devi was studying with Krishnamacharya, Iyengar was still a cowed, scrawny young man who'd been forced into yoga to earn his livelihood. Yet, in the late 1930s, Krishnamacharya sent Iyengar north to the city of Pune to teach in colleges and gymnasiums, and there, away from his fearsome master, he developed a genuine passion for the practice and grew into one of the most innovative yoga teachers in the world.

At first, Iyengar started reading about yoga in order to improve both his English and his teaching, knowing that if he failed as an instructor, he'd have to go back to Mysore. "Freedom had come to me by chance and I did not want to lose it at any cost," he writes. "If I returned, I would have to rejoin my *guruji*." He quickly realized how little consistency there was in most asana guides. "I felt that these practitioners were presenting *asana* according to their whims and fancies," he writes. So he set out to refine and standardize the asanas, developing a slow, exacting, anatomically precise style that employed props to help students perfect their alignment.

Iyengar's instruction had a profound impact on Menuhin. As he learned to relax, critics detected a new intensity and an elevated level of artistry in his playing. "In recent years there has been evidence of a struggle going on within him," wrote *New York Times* critic Howard Taubman. "Whatever private difficulties he has had with his art, he seemed to have conquered them."

Menuhin gave yoga much of the credit. In 1953, *Life* magazine did a multipage spread about his devotion to the discipline, headlined "Yehudi's Yoga," with photos of him performing various asanas and *kriyas*, or cleansing practices. In one, he's shown running a string through his nose and out his mouth, which he said helped his sense of smell and "makes his eyes bright." Another has him standing on his head. Yoga, he told the magazine, was even more important to him than violin practice. The story, in such a quintessentially mainstream publication, was further evidence that hatha yoga was moving in from the margins.

Thanks largely to Menuhin, B. K. S. Iyengar would become an international celebrity. In 1954 he summered with the violinist and his family in Gstaad. Menuhin introduced his master to the Standard Oil heiress Rebekah Harkness, who in the summer of 1956 brought him to spend six weeks in her Watch Hill, Rhode Island, mansion. Once again, *Life* ran photographs. In one, Iyengar is teaching Harkness's family to do the forward bend known as *Janu Sirsasana*, with one leg extended and the other folded into the groin. Another shows Harkness's neighbors practicing reverse prayer on her front lawn, their palms pressed together between their shoulder blades. In a third, Iyengar balances on his forearms on top of a low wall overlooking the sea, his back arched so that his feet rest on his head. The headline is "A New Twist for Society."

Yet for Americans who couldn't afford to import an Indian guru, there were still few qualified instructors. Iyengar wasn't impressed with the United States and wouldn't return until 1973. "I saw Americans were interested in the three Ws," he said later. "Wealth, women, and wine. I was taken aback to see how the way of life conflicted with my own country." The 1924 Immigration Act continued to keep other Indians from settling in the United States.

People began writing to Devi, begging for a more detailed guide to home practice, something that went beyond the overview in *Forever Young, Forever Healthy*. "Many were . . . afraid of falling into the hands of charlatans and self-appointed teachers when seeking advice, since there seems to be quite a number of unscrupulous and dishonest individuals who style themselves as real yogis, but who are only out to exploit the name of Yoga," writes Devi. She began to think about opening a center to train teachers herself. In the meantime, she started her second book, *Yoga for Americans*, designed as a complete six-week home course. It was dedicated to Gloria Swanson, "for her ever-searching, burning, crusading spirit, admirable courage, keen sense of humor and luminous laughter."

The book has a chipper, secular practicality perfectly calibrated for Eisenhower's America. (In some ways, it prefigures the contemporary literature on the business applications of mindfulness meditation.) "Yoga is of great value not only to artists engaged in creative work," Devi writes. "It will help businessmen and sportsmen, public speakers, models and housewives, and also people employed in offices, factories and stores where they must either sit at a desk, stand on their feet for long hours at a time, or work under stresses and tensions."

Menuhin penned the foreword. "This welcome book by Indra Devi is further evidence of the interest that has been awakened in the United States, Canada, and other countries of the Western world, for the practical aspects, applicable to our own mode of living, of the ancient science of yoga," he wrote.

Like her first book, *Yoga for Americans* was an enormous success. People started calling Devi the First Lady of Yoga. As Menuhin suggested, yoga was catching on all over the world, not just in the United States. *Forever Young, Forever Healthy* had been translated into a number of languages, including French, German, Spanish, Portuguese, and Italian. One reader of the Japanese edition (thought to be the first book about yoga published in that country) wrote to Devi from Osaka to thank her for alleviating his nervous heart condition, his wife's weight problem, and his son's asthma. A letter from a German fan read, "The Yoga exercises are remarkable: The fat ones get slimmer and the thin ones gain weight and get stronger; constipation disappears, the body becomes elastic and the spirits brighten up."

Devi even managed to bring her message to Russia. A June 1960 United Press International dispatch from Moscow announced her triumph with the headline "Red Heads Turn for Yankee Yogi."

"Yoga has been introduced to Kremlin leaders—head stands and all—by a woman teacher from Hollywood," read the story. Devi had taken her first trip back to the Soviet Union since fleeing the Russian Revolution as a teenager, and she'd brought her yoga with her. Given that most spiritual practices were outlawed in the USSR, this was something of a coup.

Details of this remarkable journey are spotty, but we know that it was K. P. S. Menon, Devi's old friend from China, who arranged the gathering with the Kremlin bigwigs. He had since become ambassador to the USSR, and when Devi, traveling with a student of hers in northern Europe, wanted to visit her old homeland, she turned to him for help. It's not clear how the idea came about, but that summer, with the Cold War raging and the Soviet Union still very much cut off from the Western world, Devi managed to get papers and visit the country of her youth for the first time in more than forty years. Her student, whom she refers to as Bala Krishna but otherwise says little about, accompanied her.

She arrived in Leningrad after giving a lecture in Oslo. Much of it was unrecognizable, though the house where she'd lived with her grandmother when the city was called St. Petersburg still stood. In Moscow she checked in to the once-grand Hotel Metropol, where she'd stayed with her mother as a girl. People gawked at her as she walked the streets in her sari, stopping her to ask where she was from and why she was there.

According to a story she later told, a young man noticed one of her yoga books under her bag at a restaurant and begged her to sell it to him; at the time, books about Eastern religions were available only on the black market. She gave him the book and even offered to teach him a deep-breathing technique, though they had a hard time finding a place where they could be alone. The streets were too crowded, and he knew better than to go to a foreigner's hotel. Finally, they hid in a quiet corner of a subway station, but Devi had to cut the lesson short when a suspicious soldier started watching them. "The prospect of being questioned at a police station did not particularly appeal to me," she writes. "It would have been rather difficult to explain why an American citizen, dressed in an Indian sari, would want to show a strange Russian youth the Yoga method of deep breathing—and in a subway station at that!"

Despite the oppressive atmosphere, Devi never really expressed any anger toward the Soviet system that had turned her and her mother into refugees. This wasn't, contrary to the Red-hunters' suspicions, due to any sort of leftist impulse. Rather, it was a product of her determined political detachment, a result of both her otherworldly inclinations and her spiritual discipline. Once, she recalls in her memoir, some students in Paris were discomfited by her refusal to condemn the Bolsheviks. "They weren't interested in talking with someone who simply accepted things as they were and decided to live her life free from historical conflicts," she writes. For someone who'd been buffeted by global cataclysm the way she had, part of yoga's power was its promise of an escape from history, a way to remain impervious to life's daily chaos and contingency.

While Devi had no interest in communism, she was happy for the chance to bring yoga to Communists. She got her chance when Menon arranged a reception for her attended by top Soviet officials, including First Deputy Premier Anastas Mikoyan (the second-most powerful figure in the country, next to Nikita Khrushchev) and Foreign Minister Andrei Gromyko. Devi, the only woman in the large hall, stood on a small platform covered with carpets and plants and, speaking in Russian, gave a brief overview of hatha yoga. Her student Bala Krishna demonstrated a few postures.

When she was finished, the assembled dignitaries peppered her with questions. Their interest wasn't as odd as it might seem—while the Soviet Union was hostile to religion, there was a lot of official interest in what was called "human reserves," hidden potentials that might somehow be unleashed for the benefit of the state. During the late 1950s, as a result of rumors that American researchers were conducting telepathy experiments aboard submarines, there was a burst of Soviet research into parapsychology, including a brief period of openness to Western experts. Starting in 1963, reported the British magazine *New Scientist*, "Numerous Western researchers travelled to Russia and found a fair amount of activity and interest in the paranormal, although the focus was frequently different from that in the West. Russian workers tended to be far more preoccupied with physical and biological effects than with the so-called 'mental' phenomena of telepathy and clairvoyance."

Not surprisingly, researchers into human reserves were particularly interested in the feats of Indian yogis. Searching for ways that cosmonauts could control their physiological processes in space, a scientist named A. S. Romen spent several years researching yoga methods before developing a technique called "self-regulation," essentially Sovietized hatha yoga. It began with deep relaxation in which practitioners would breathe rhythmically while attempting to release all muscular tension. Then they would, through the power of concentration, try to raise and lower their body temperatures and manipulate the rhythm of their heartbeats, just like advanced yogis. Afterward, they would breathe deeply and do simple stretching exercises. Some of Romen's subjects learned to perform yogic abdominal contractions while seated in the lotus position.

So, Russian authorities would have been open to Devi's message, as long as they were convinced she was promoting a useful technology rather than a form of irrational mysticism. Was yoga, Mikoyan asked, a religion? No, Devi assured him. Yoga helps people develop their full physical, spiritual, and mental potentials; it could be practiced by people of any faith or none.

Yet the word *spirit* made Mikoyan uneasy. What was the difference between that and religion? In Devi's telling, she countered by asking whether Tolstoy had a highly developed spirit.

"Tolstoy is a spiritual giant!" Mikoyan exclaimed.

Yet, she argued, he was refused a religious burial. "A spiritual giant is not always a religious person, and a religious person doesn't always have a developed spirit," she said. This seems to have convinced Mikoyan, since, as she told it, he approached the platform, held out his hand, and helped her climb down. Foreign Minister Gromkyo offered a vodka toast.

For ordinary Russians who aspired to become yogis, Devi's overtures to the Soviet leadership didn't necessarily make things any easier. In the years after her visit, yoga books, including *Forever Young, Forever Healthy*, were illicitly translated, photocopied, and distributed by hand, and underground clubs devoted to yoga and other New Age practices proliferated, but the discipline was frowned upon and could get practitioners into trouble. A *New York Times* dispatch from 1973 headlined "Yoga Exercise Fad in Soviet Is Vigorously Attacked" quoted a meeting of athletic officials who had denounced yoga for doing nothing for "the development of active working people" and for being an "idealistic philosophy full of mysticism." In the 1980s, some Russian yoga teachers were still ending up in prison.

Yet, three years after Devi's trip, Dhirendra Brahmachari, yoga teacher to the Nehru family, traveled to Russia to train Soviet cosmonauts. (Years later, Brahmachari would come to be known as the "Indian Rasputin" because of his malign influence on Indira Gandhi.) In the Soviet Union, as in the United States, there was room for yoga as long as it was grounded in secular materialism, its mysticism pulsing just under the surface, waiting until the time was right to show itself.

By 1960, anticommunist paranoia had calmed down enough that somehow the FBI, which had stopped following Devi and questioning her friends and students, didn't notice her trip. At least, no mention of it appears in her file until 1962, when she landed on the Bureau's radar again due to a tip by a suspicious woman named Doris Jean Hollenbeck.

Hollenbeck worked in newspaper promotion and advertising, and her husband, from whom she was separated, was a colonel in the Marine Corps. She met Devi at a luncheon, and Devi, ever eager to enlist new acquaintances in her plans, thought Hollenbeck might be able to help her promote the use of yoga in American factories and in the military, which she believed would improve well-being and efficiency. She invited Hollenbeck to visit her at home, and Hollenbeck went.

The newspaper woman, wrote an FBI agent, "was of the opinion that she was 'being sounded out' to determine her personal attitude toward Russia. During the course of the visit, DEVI brought out that she is the daughter of a former Czarist General Officer. DEVI indicated no displeasure with the current Russian Regime. She talked of the use of Yoga by Russian industry, Russian military forces, Russian Cosmonauts, etc."

Hollenbeck's apprehension didn't stop her from visiting Devi several more times, either because she was intrigued or because she wanted to gather more information. During a subsequent get-together, she overheard Devi and her husband discussing Devi's travel to the Soviet Union, and noted to the FBI that she was "favorably inclined" to the trip. (It's not clear if the conversation she overheard was about the 1960 journey or about plans for a future one.)

"Mrs. HOLLENBECK said DEVI and her husband are part of an International Set," reported the FBI agent. Hollenbeck had, she admitted, "no information that would indicate DEVI is trying to use her program to the detriment of the United States." Yet, the report said, reviewing Devi's books and recordings, Hollenbeck had concluded "that the material is soporific in nature and that it could be part of a program to be used against the U.S."

This might have been the start of a new round of surveillance, but the FBI seems to have lost interest, perhaps because agents believed Devi had relocated to Mexico, where she and Knauer bought a villa in 1960. (One memo written in response to Hollenbeck's claims notes that Devi was in Mexico and says, "No further investigation in this case is contemplated at Los Angeles.")

Devi had fallen in love with Mexico while visiting the heiress Gloria Gasque, former president of the International Vegetarian Union, at her home in Tecate, a town directly over the border. Tecate had a lovely, arid, Mediterranean climate and had been spared the tawdry tourist invasion that had transformed Tijuana, twenty-five miles to the west. Gasque had built a three-story house with sixteen bedrooms at the foot of a mountain that the Americans called Tecate Peak and the Mexicans referred to as Mount Cuchuma. Rancho Cuchuma, as Gasque had named her estate, was surrounded by an organic vegetable garden and a small stand of fruit trees; inside the house were splendid oriental rugs, tapestries, and crystal chandeliers. It seemed to Devi like an exotic and refined palace, the sort of place she had lived in many years before in India.

Next door to Gasque's house was Rancho La Puerta, a world-famous health spa. The owners, Deborah and Edmond Szekely, had founded it in 1940 as part health camp, part commune—at first, everyone had to bring his own tent, chop firewood, and perform farm chores. Edmond Szekely, a world-traveling polyglot Hungarian shaped by *Lebensreform*, was an early evangelist for whole, organic food, and much of what he and his wife served came from their garden: fresh raw milk from their goats, wild sage honey, sprouted wheat, salads, and tropical fruits.

Initially, the camp was called the Essene School of Life. The name was based on Szekely's claim that an ancient Aramaic manuscript hidden in the Vatican Library, the Essene Gospel of Peace, revealed Jesus as a prophet of vegetarianism, fresh air, and health fasts. Soon, word got out that a visit to the Essene School of Life was a great way to lose weight, and a new sort of guest started showing up: women who wanted to be pampered while they searched for the keys to eternal youth.

The Szekelys changed the name of their retreat to the less metaphysical Rancho La Puerta. Deborah added calisthenics classes, dance classes, hydrotherapy, herbal wraps, and other beauty treatments. Naturally, they needed a hatha yoga teacher. So when Gasque died, the Szekelys suggested that Devi buy Rancho Cuchuma. Knauer put up the money, and in 1962, Devi opened a yoga school where she would train a generation of teachers to meet the burgeoning American demand.

The nature of that demand was quickly changing. The United States was on the verge of the Age of Aquarius, when huge numbers of spiritually parched Americans would turn eastward, seeking not just health but also transcendence. As they did so, Devi would cast off the air of industrious pragmatism that had, until then, served her so well in Los Angeles and Moscow alike. Yoga in the West was about to get a lot more ecstatic and wild, and Devi, who never really gave up her quest for a guru, was about to find a brand-new god.

T'S NOT CLEAR what Devi expected to get out of her madly impractical trip to Saigon in 1966, when the Vietnam War was raging. In her writings and interviews, she says only that she went there to conduct meditations. The trip was part of a grand but amorphous project called the Crusade for Light in Darkness, which Devi began in 1965, but because it never really came to fruition, she didn't write much about it. It's likely that she was pulled to Vietnam by the same centripetal force that always drew her to the spinning center of things; even as she professed a desire to live outside history, there was a part of her that loved being close to the action. She'd had success in the past with impulsive leaps into foreign lands and barely constructed plans that somehow seemed to work out, and she had faith that wherever she went, even a country at war, the universe would ensure her well-being.

The idea for the Crusade arose during a fateful trip to Dallas in November 1963. Devi had quite a following in the city thanks to Elsie Frankfurt, who, along with her sisters, had founded Page Boy, the country's first line of fashionable, upscale maternity clothes. Frankfurt, a millionaire and a minor celebrity, had met Devi while vacationing at Rancho La Puerta and been so impressed that she instituted daily yoga breaks for all employees in her Dallas factory, bringing Devi to town that spring to help start the program. Over two days, Devi went from department to department, offering individual instruction in deep breathing and restorative asanas, and then leading the whole office through relaxation exercises over the loudspeaker.

After her visit, every day at 1:55 p.m., switchboard operators at the factory would interrupt all calls to announce, "[Y]oga break starts at 2!" When the hour struck, the entire factory shuddered to a halt. Buyers in the showroom were told they could either wait or join in as Elsie or one of her sisters used the loudspeaker to lead the session. "The elevators are motionless and the porters lay down their mops," reported the *New York Herald Tribune.* "Since there aren't enough mats yet to go around, some of the employees stretch out on the floor and others push aside the maternity dresses and lie down on the cutting tables, while they breathe deep and perfect their yoga." The story also noted that Frankfurt was planning to make yoga clothes—what she called a "lotus suit"—for expectant mothers, prefiguring the prenatal yoga boom by several decades.

Because of Frankfurt, the *Herald Tribune* reported, yoga was "running rampant" in Dallas. So it was a natural place for Devi to stop while on tour for her latest book, *Renew Your Life through Yoga,* which describes how yoga offers release from anxiety, the "Problem of Our Age" and "one of the greatest menaces the civilized world must face these days." When she realized that she was going to be in the city at the same time as President John F. Kennedy—whose iconic wife, Jackie, had worn Page Boy attire during her pregnancies—she hoped to meet him and possibly teach him some deep-breathing exercises that he might use to cope with the enormous strain of his job.

He was dead before she got the chance. Kennedy's assassination shocked her deeply and seems to have awakened in her some of the religious hunger she'd put aside during the years of her great American success. Like much of the emerging counterculture, she was becoming convinced that the world was in the midst of a spiritual crisis, one that yoga and meditation could perhaps help to solve.

Thus, after years of trying to persuade Westerners that yoga had nothing to do with religion, she suddenly found herself ready for a divine quest.

The details of that quest, though, never quite got nailed down. Part of the plan was to build what she called a "Tower of Light" in Tecate, with an eternal flame that she would carry from country to country like an Olympic torch. This would be followed by a series of mass meditations held in stadiums in which people would "attempt to stir the 'forces of light' into action to combat the 'forces of darkness' so active in this day and age," she told the *New Cosmic Star*, a monthly New Age newspaper. "We will stress the performance of acts of kindness, light and goodness . . . keep your heart clean, be extraordinarily kind." Afterward, all participants would light a candle from the eternal flame and keep it burning in their windows until the end of the Crusade.

In April 1965, everyone in Devi's address book received a typed fund-raising letter suggesting that they honor her sixty-sixth birthday by making a donation toward the project. "On May 12, her birthday, INDRA DEVI will start on a 'CRUSADE FOR LIGHT IN DARKNESS,' believing that this will bring LIGHT into the lives of thousands and possibly millions because she wants to spend the rest of her life on this CRUSADE," it read. "Without adequate assistance, without proper organization and necessary funds, this COURAGEOUS LITTLE WOMAN who is always full of enthusiasm, always ready to help others has decided to start on this CRUSADE because she says, 'the call is so persistent that she cannot disobey it and will just go ahead believing angels and men will come to help.'"

The Crusade kicked off at a ceremony on May 8, when the mayors of Tecate and nearby National City, California, joined her to lay the Tower's foundation stone at Rancho Cuchuma. There was another ceremony on May 12 at National City's Kimball Community Hall. That year, she released a vinyl record, *Indra Devi Presents Concentration & Meditation*, whose cover described her as "The World's Foremost Authority on Yoga" and the "Founder of the Crusade for Light in Darkness." Its front featured a portrait of Devi by the Dallas artist Dmitri Vail, known for his expensive paintings of socialites, celebrities, and politicians. She's shown in a white sari with a sort of silver Renaissance halo behind her head. Eyes cast heavenward, she stands before what appears to be an altar and holds a small oil lamp in her hands, like an offering. Never before had she presented herself in such an overtly spiritual guise.

On the recording, which is less than a half-hour long, her voice is melodious and almost girlish as she instructs listeners to summon their inner light through visualization and concentration, and then to direct it outward, toward those they love as well as those they hate. She enlists her audience in a cosmic spiritual struggle, saying, "Those who are on the dark side are very active. They're violent, they're loud, they kill . . . and what are you doing, if you are on the side of light? You cannot just do nothing." As she presents it, meditation becomes both a way of letting go of the world and of improving it.

Nothing more seems to have happened with the crusade until 1966, when Devi traveled to India "carrying the fire of peace and solidarity," which she planned to present to Prime Minister Indira Gandhi, daughter of her old friend Jawaharlal Nehru, on behalf of the women of Mexico.

Bringing a fire across the globe by commercial airplane, it turned out, wasn't easy. After starting the flame with a magnifying glass atop Mount Cuchuma, Devi was determined not to extinguish it, lest she undermine the symbolism of her pilgrimage. Yet even in 1966, when airline security was far more lax than it is today, you couldn't get on a plane with a burning candle. So, as she prepared to board a flight to New York for the first leg of the trip, she devised a clever solution. She used the fire to light some incense, which she somehow smuggled aboard in the folds of her sari and then hid in an ashtray. On the plane, she used the incense to light a cigarette, which, with the help of some obliging fellow passengers, was then used to light others throughout the flight. When the plane was to land and the No Smoking sign switched on, Devi hid one of the lit cigarettes in her ashtray, then used it to light yet another cigarette when the plane touched down.

"I assure you, I did not rest until we lit a match from this cigarette when we got to the hotel and then lit a large candle from this match," she told the *New Cosmic Star*. She repeated this process on a flight from New York to Rome, where she carried the flame to the Vatican and somehow, she said, arranged to have Pope Paul VI bless it. From there, she went to Delhi, where Indira Gandhi had just, months before, been installed as prime minister following the death of the country's previous leader, Lal Bahadur Shastri. A newspaper photo captured the ceremony during which Devi handed a lotus-shaped vessel containing the flame to Gandhi. The Indian leader appeared reverent, her eyes downcast and her head covered by her sari. The caption noted that, from India, the flame was to be "taken all over the world."

It was an extravagantly crazy idea to bring the Crusade to Vietnam, though there was also a certain logic to it. Devi was still deeply apolitical and never took a public stance on the war itself, but you didn't have to be an activist to recognize that much of the world's turmoil was distilled in that country. She doesn't seem to have had a plan in place for what would happen when she got there, but she was used to charging into the unknown and having it work out. Perhaps she thought that when she arrived, men and angels would lead her to her next step.

On the way to Saigon, Devi stopped in Madras to see an old friend from her Theosophy days, a doctor named Sivakamu. (She was the elder sister of Rukmini Devi Arundale, whom Annie Besant had once come close to declaring the World Mother.) Devi decided to stay at the Adyar Theosophical headquarters, revisiting the tranquil, leafy estate where she'd first landed in India almost forty years earlier. It was just supposed to be a brief detour, but there, once again, people were buzzing about a new Indian messiah, and for Devi, learning about him would change everything.

Devi first heard the name Sai Baba from Howard Murphet and his wife, Iris, Australian Theosophists in late middle age who had come to India searching for divinity. As it happens, Howard's fascination with yoga philosophy had been piqued while he was studying at the Sydney yoga studio of Michael Volin, Devi's former assistant in Shanghai. Eventually, he and his wife decided to come to India in the hope of lapping up spiritual wisdom at its source.

"Was there, we wondered, anything left of the mysterious India described in the pages of Paul Brunton, Yogananda, Kipling, Madame Blavatsky, Colonel H. S. Olcott and other writers?" Murphet writes. "Were there still hidden fountains of esoteric knowledge or had the ancient springs dried up?" He and Iris began their quest by enrolling in a six-month "School of the Wisdom" at the Theosophical Society, after which they traveled the country seeking audiences with various gurus and holy men.

They met the Dalai Lama, not yet an international celebrity, in Dharamsala, the Himalayan town where he lived in exile. They visited the Sivananda ashram in Rishikesh, discoursed with cave-dwelling sadhus, and met the Maharishi Mahesh Yogi, who, thanks to the Beatles, would soon become a global superstar. Sai Baba, though, had captivated them above all others. "He seemed to lift us up to some high level where there were no more worries," Murphet writes of his first encounter with the guru. "Life became larger than life, and the usual difficulties and conflicts of the mundane world were far off, unreal. There seemed to be an aura of happiness around us. Iris mentioned that she could not stop herself smiling for hours after Baba had talked to her."

"He is the brightest star in the spiritual firmament of India today," Howard told Devi. "He is an Avatar, a Divine Incarnation."

"You must . . . you simply must meet him," added Iris.

Devi, however, wasn't interested. When they showed her his picture—"a fat, fierce-looking man in a bright orange robe," with a nimbus of wiry hair like an afro—all she could say was "Why this wild hairdo?" Sai Baba was due to arrive in Madras, and the Murphets urged Devi to wait, but she was eager to continue her Crusade and disappointed them by leaving for Vietnam as planned.

In Saigon, she stayed with the Indian consul general. She told Natalia Apostolli, her biographer, that she conducted candlelight meditations in various temples and pagodas, but aside from that, no record exists of the weeks she spent in the city. In some ways it must have recalled her days in Shanghai and, before that, Berlin, with their strange mix of violence, terror, and antic gaiety. There were frequent Vietcong bombings. Protests against the South Vietnamese military junta were beaten back by riot police, leaving the streets full of teargas. The sound of artillery rumbled through the night, searchlights strafed the Saigon River, and fighter planes and jet bombers roared as they took off from Tan Son Nhat airport.

At the same time, the city throbbed with life. "Saigon swings," the Associated Press's Hugh Mulligan wrote around the period Devi arrived. "The streets are full of flowers and thronged with women shoppers, wearing the colorful form-fitting ow-dais [sic], until a bomb erupts and everyone scatters. German acrobats and Spanish flamenco dancers and Greek snake charmers and all sorts of other exotic acts from what surely must be the bottom of the vaudeville barrel perform in smoky nightclubs now crowded with American soldiers." Such apocalyptic festivity, so strange to most people, would have been familiar to Devi.

Yet what was she doing there? It's hard to imagine who in Vietnam she might have passed her sacred flame to. When six U.S. pacifists visited Saigon that spring, young anticommunists pelted them with eggs and tomatoes. There was mounting anti-Americanism among the organized Buddhists, who opposed the U.S.-supported regime and would almost certainly have been suspicious of overtures from a white-haired Western lady of indeterminate accent. The city was tense and complicated and full of conspiracy, and even as lucky and charismatic a woman as Devi could not blithely show up and expect any sort of welcome.

Whatever happened, she never wrote about the trip except in

passing, as a detail in the story of how she found Sai Baba. For it was in Saigon, she writes, that a desire to meet him took hold, soon growing so intense that after a couple of weeks she decided to return to India early. Perhaps, in the sudden desire to see the guru, she was able to imbue a failed trip with meaning. Her roundabout route to him proved that the universe was watching out for her after all.

According to legend, shortly after Sathya Sai Baba was born on November 23, 1926, in a parched, remote Indian village called Puttaparthi, he was placed on a blanket that started, mysteriously, to move. There was a cobra beneath it, but it didn't harm the boy. This was seen as remarkably auspicious, the cobra being a symbol of Shiva. From the beginning, the child was marked as divine.

By the time the boy—then known as Satyanarayana Raju, or Sathya, for short—was in elementary school, he was known for playful little miracles, producing, for instance, handfuls of sweets from an empty bag for other children. He played magical pranks, such as freezing a teacher to his chair. At thirteen, possibly following a scorpion's bite, he went through an agonizing spiritual crisis, becoming, for a time, terrifyingly erratic. "He seldom answered when spoken to; he had little interest in food; he would suddenly burst into song or poetry, sometimes quoting long Sanskrit passages far beyond anything learned in his formal education and training," writes Murphet. "Off and on he would become stiff, appearing to leave his body and go somewhere else."

Believing the boy possessed by evil spirits, Sathya's terrified parents brought him to an exorcist, who tried to drive away the incorporeal interlopers by torturing the body they were living in. The fearsome demon-fighter shaved the boy's head; sliced deep, bloody crosses on his skull; and poured lime and garlic into the wounds. He dumped 108 pots of cold water over him, beat him on his joints, and rubbed a searing acid mixture into his eyes. Eventually, Sathya's parents couldn't stand it anymore and took their unchanged son away.

They tried other doctors and healers, but no one could do anything to fix the strange, unstable child.

Then, his biographers say, after about two months of bizarre behavior, Sathya called his family members around him and, in a joyful mood, started materializing sugar candy and flowers with a wave of his hand. Neighbors crowded in, and the smiling boy plucked treats for them from the air—more candy and flowers, as well as rice balls cooked in milk. His father had been tending to his produce store while all this was going on, and when he heard what was happening, he was furious, convinced that his son was either fooling everyone with sleight of hand or, worse, using black magic. "This is too much! It must stop! What are you?" Sathya's father asked. "Tell me—a ghost, or a god, or a madcap?"

"I am Sai Baba," the boy replied.

Sai Baba had been the name of a deceased holy man from a town called Shirdi in the Indian state of Maharashtra. He was famous for combining Hindu and Sufi Muslim forms of devotion, and for preaching the unity of all religions in a country often convulsed by sectarianism. He lived in a dilapidated mosque and had a reputation as a miracle worker; ash from a sacred fire that he kept burning at all times was used as a cure for manifold ailments. Sai Baba of Shirdi had died in 1918. Now young Satyanarayana Raju insisted that he was this man's reincarnation.

His parents continued to doubt him, but the boy's following grew. A bouquet of jasmine was said to have spelled out "Sai Baba" when he scattered it on the floor. He produced photos of Shirdi Sai Baba with a wave of his hand and plucked dates and flowers from the air—offerings, he said, that had been left at the shrine of his previous body. Despite all this, his parents insisted he go back to school, and for a while he complied, until one day in 1940 he threw away his books and announced that he was leaving. "My devotees are calling me. I have my work," he said.

After that he lived with followers, and wherever he was, worshippers would gather to sing *bhajans*, or devotional songs. People began to arrive from nearby towns and villages, and from Bangalore, one hundred miles away, to see the miraculous young man, now known as Sathya Sai Baba, or simply Sai Baba. Barely five feet tall, he had frizzy black hair that stood straight up from his head, a pudgy face, and soft, dark eyes overflowing with both compassion and mischief. His charisma was powerful but also effervescent; he loved jokes and preached a gospel of love. For devotees, simply being in his presence conferred blessings.

Sathya Sai Baba began to attract an elite following, including members of the royal families of Mysore, Sandur, Venkatagiri, and Chincholi, as well as landlords, government officials, and wealthy businessmen. In 1945 his devotees built him a temple at the edge of his village, and in 1950 it was expanded into an ashram called Prasanthi Nilayam, or "Abode of Supreme Peace."

During those early years, his following was still small enough to be intimate. In the dry season, he'd take devotees to the sands of the Chitravathi River to sing and discuss matters of the spirit. "We'd sit there and talk, just a few of us, like a family, close and full of love," one of his acolytes, a woman doctor, told the screenwriter Arnold Schulman, who published an admiring, enigmatic book about Sai Baba in 1971. "He'd start playing with the sand, pouring it from one hand to another the way a child does, and all of a sudden as the sand fell from one hand to the other you could see it turn into a ring or a necklace or a statue of Krishna."

Other early devotees told stories of "wish-fulfilling trees" that, by Sai Baba's grace, would yield any fruit they named. He cured illnesses and made food multiply. "At picnics he would tap empty dishes, and when the lids were removed, the dishes would be full of food, sometimes hot as if straight from the kitchen," one of his followers told Murphet. Miracles, he often said, were his calling card, his way of gathering people around him and opening them to his message, which was about the oneness of all faiths and the need to love God in whatever form you envisioned Him. He was like a jolly Jesus, and his followers had the ecstatic sense that they were modern-day apostles, supporting players in a world-transforming drama.

In 1963, Sai Baba made an announcement: he was not just a guru, but an avatar, the living incarnation of the god Shiva and the goddess Shakti, a being in which the male and female aspects of the divine reach a sacred unity. The first Sai Baba, he said, had incarnated the male Shiva alone. He prophesied a third incarnation, Prema Sai, who would appear after his death and incarnate Shakti. (In some versions of the Sai gospel, the incarnations are reversed, with Sai Baba of Shirdi embodying the goddess, and the future Prema Sai the god.) What was significant was not just Sai Baba assuming the mantle of a celestial androgyny or positing himself as part of a holy trinity. It was his claim that he wasn't simply here to lead people to God. He *was* God.

After she met him, Indra Devi would, for a time, come to agree.

Returning to India from Vietnam, Devi first went to Adyar, where she got a letter of introduction from the Murphets. From there, she headed three hundred miles inland, to Mysore, where, courtesy of a princess named Rani Vijaya Devi, she was put up at the palace where she'd lived while studying with Krishnamacharya. Then, packing just enough for a few days, she hired a car for the bumpy two-hundred-mile drive to the ashram.

The final hours of the trip were jarring, as the car jerked along a dirt track through barren, red-clay countryside, stopping whenever animals wandered in front of it. It was April, the height of summer in the region, when temperatures regularly climbed past one hundred degrees Fahrenheit.

Finally, they arrived in the desiccated South Indian town where Sai Baba was born. The ashram was on Puttaparthi's outskirts and had become the center of its economy. On the dusty road to Prasanthi Nilayam's main gate, makeshift stalls catered to a constant stream of pilgrims, offering photographs of Sai Baba and rings and buttons bearing his image. Dozens of women sat in the dirt peddling shriveled produce. Beggars, some with maimed or deformed children, put out their hands for alms.

Inside the brick wall that enclosed the ashram, things were more orderly. Rows of coconut palms lined the path to a spacious, white-washed prayer hall, built in a vaguely Mughal style. It was the center of ashram life, and Sai Baba lived above it. Most Indian visitors camped out in enormous open tin-roof sheds, where up to two hundred people would sleep end to end on the floor and cook on small kerosene stoves. Westerners and upper-class Indians who were accustomed to greater comforts were put up in a spartan guesthouse, and that's where Devi was assigned a room. There was a list of rules on the veranda. One of them forbade giving donations or gifts to Sai Baba, even customary offerings such as fruit or flowers. This was highly unusual for an Indian ashram, and it impressed Devi. Would a fraud refuse to let people give him money?

A young Swiss woman named Gabriella Steyer, one of Sai Baba's earliest Western acolytes, met Devi and showed her around. They visited the small hospital, the only one for miles, which was built by Baba's devotees and offered care for free. Though there were two doctors on staff, Baba was said to intervene in cases where medical treatment wasn't enough, and the ashram buzzed with stories of remarkable, inexplicable cures. Steyer took Devi to the Veda-Shastra School, where boys studied religious texts, learning to chant the Vedas by heart, a project that could take twenty years. Tuition was free, said Steyer, and Baba gave students food, lodging, and clothes. There was a small press that produced a monthly ashram magazine in English and Telugu, the local language, as well as a post office, a bank, a police station, and a canteen staffed by volunteers.

Back in Devi's room, Steyer regaled her with stories of Baba's miracles. She recalled a holiday when Baba led the ashramites to a river outside the village and, after drawing on the sand with his finger, reached in and pulled out a silver idol, a chalice, and a spoon. He then squeezed heavenly nectar out of his closed fist, filling the chalice with it, and giving each of his devotees a delicious spoonful. Each time it ran out, he tapped the chalice to fill it again.

Devi was not yet convinced, but she was eager to meet the man said to work such wonders. Finally, Steyer took her to the prayer hall, where Baba was speaking privately with some of his devotees in a room set apart for such meetings. A side door opened to let some people out, and Devi got her first sight of the guru. Draped in a saffron-colored robe, he was slight despite his full face and more handsome than she expected—he looked hardly at all like the coarse-featured man in the Murphets' photograph. His bristly hair seemed to form a black halo around his head, and he appeared divinely gentle, glowing with compassion. He said a few words in Telugu and disappeared. Someone translated: "No more interviews—it is too late."

A few minutes later, though, Baba appeared on the balcony outside his apartment, surveying the crowd below. His eyes met Devi's, and she felt sure he was going to summon her. Her heart started pounding. Sure enough, in what felt like an instant, he was standing in front of her, beckoning her into the room where he held his private audiences. As she walked toward him, she felt as if she were floating. Steyer and a few other women, who had also been invited, had to hold her up.

Sai Baba had an armchair in the room, but he took a seat opposite Devi on the floor. She told him she didn't know why she was there—she'd heard his name for the first time only a few weeks before, and she didn't need anything from him. "It was in Saigon that suddenly I was overcome by a desire to see you," she said.

He asked her where she was from, and she showed him a picture of Rancho Cuchuma. "You must come there, Swamiji—it is a beautiful place," she said. He took her hand and promised that he would, repeating it three times.

Then, looking at the sleeve where she kept the photo, he noticed that she also had a picture of Swami Vivekananda. She told him that she believed Vivekananda was her protector and guardian angel and that he must have guided her steps to Prasanthi Nilayam. "You would not be here otherwise," he said.

As they parted, he asked her, "What do you want?" She had been told to expect the question. "Jyoti," she replied. "Light. Light in my heart."

"You have it," he said.

"Not enough."

"Bangaru, bangaru," he said, a Telugu endearment. He told her he was going to give her something to keep with her during meditation. Turning his palm down, he made a circling motion. When he flipped his hand over, he held a little enamel image of himself, which he put into her hand. She was astonished and didn't doubt the authenticity of what she had witnessed.

"Wait," he said. "Let me also give you some *vibhuti*." That was the name for the sacred ash that was Baba's signature, a substance that linked him in some mysterious way to Shirdi Sai Baba and his ever-burning fire. Devi writes that he poured the *vibhuti* from his fingertips until it covered the image in her hand. Then he took the icon and the ash and wrapped it in a piece of paper.

"Call me whenever you need me, I shall hear you no matter what the distance," he told her. "I am yours."

She was overwhelmed, dazed, and ecstatic. Sai Baba had a way of making the world seem enchanted, as if the magic that filled ancient religious books could also pervade modern life. Devi had never stopped hungering for such rapture, even if she'd stopped actively seeking it after Krishnamurti. Now here she was at sixty-seven, as filled with spiritual excitement as she was in Ommen forty years earlier.

At five o'clock the next morning, Devi joined hundreds of other devotees to await *darshan*, the ritual in which Sai Baba allowed his acolytes to gaze upon him and feel the blessing of his presence. Life in the ashram, she quickly discovered, revolved around *darshan*— Bill Aitken, one of Baba's biographers, calls it the "both the central communion and the theology of the movement." As she walked toward the temple, the echoing sound of "Om" floated toward her from devotees who had already assembled. Two hours passed, anticipation mounting.

Then, finally, Sai Baba appeared outside his apartment on the second-story balcony and raised his hand in benediction. In the audience, a few lucky ones felt his eyes meet theirs, and bliss surged through them. Hope for such a moment was part of what kept them coming back, morning after morning, for the same wait and the same brief appearance. "Away from Sai's presence," writes Aitken, "our imperfection is almost too painful to behold, hence the provision of photographs, medallions and other seemingly trivial mementos of Sai Baba . . . hence, too, the discipline of sitting long hours in Puttaparthi, building up the longing of the heart for its moment of re-contact with the divine."

Devi couldn't return the next morning—she'd planned on staying only a couple of days, and she had to begin her journey home, but she felt changed by her short time in Sai Baba's orbit. Back at the Mysore Palace, she absentmindedly packed her things, forgetting many of them in the drawers. From there, she went to Bombay, where she stayed with Enakshi Bhavnani, another old friend from the Theosophical Society.

As she prepared to go back to Tecate, she found herself growing despondent, just as she had when she left India after her rapturous first visit. It had been many years since she'd felt that way, and it unnerved her. How could she return home and lecture about the transcendent peace to be found in yoga when she herself was unhappy and unsettled? She began writing Sai Baba a letter asking for his help, and then put it in her handbag while she and Bhavnani went shopping.

Suddenly, she writes, while the two of them stood on a street corner waiting for a taxi, her sadness disappeared and she felt a flood of inexpressible joy, as if a "cascade of brilliant light" were pouring over her. Convinced that Sai Baba had answered her letter before she even finished writing it, she was flooded by the same sort of bliss she'd once experienced after meeting Krishnamurti, but this time, she'd found a guru who accepted the role.

Almost as soon as she got home, Devi started making plans to return to Prasanthi Nilayam. Howard Murphet recommended that she go for the Maha Shivarathri festival, a great all-night celebration of Shiva and a holiday when Sai Baba was known to perform public miracles. The festival is held during the dark night of the new moon in the middle of the Indian month of Magha, which in 1967 fell in early March. Devi arranged to arrive a month before.

At the ashram, she heard new stories almost every day about Sai Baba's miracles. Most devotees believed that the guru spoke to them in their dreams, and so they eagerly discussed and analyzed their visions of the night before, looking for divine direction. Devi heard miraculous tales of healing and clairvoyance. The Maharani of Jind came to her room one day bubbling with excitement to tell her that Sai Baba had given her daughter, who was engaged to be married, a necklace of diamonds and pearls. "You have no father, so I am taking his place and giving you something befitting your status as a princess," he told the maharani's daughter.

A pearl fell off the necklace, but this didn't lead anyone to question the piece's value. Instead, Devi recalled the story of a man who started wondering about the monetary worth of a gold medallion Sai Baba had given him. As a result of his greed, the medallion vanished from its box. Then, when the man fell to his knees and begged for forgiveness, Baba returned it. The missing pearl was likewise taken as one of Sai Baba's playful reminders to his devotees about what truly mattered.

As the festival of Shivarathri approached, more and more people arrived at the ashram. The sheds filled up quickly, so newcomers slept under trees. When there were no more spots near the trees, they unfurled their bedrolls in the open air. By the day of the festival, around thirty thousand people had crammed into Prasanthi Nilayam. That morning, Sai Baba hoisted the ashram's flag over the temple, telling the ashramites to hoist the flag of love in their hearts. "Practice Yoga, or the mastery of the mind," he said. "Then the lotus of the heart will bloom, and illumination be attained."

He spoke of the significance of Shivarathri. The waning of the moon was associated with the waning of the mind, whose constant restless whirling and unending cacophony of desires obscured the apprehension of God. Shiva, destroyer of illusions, revealed to man his true, sacred nature. The day devoted to him was a uniquely auspicious occasion for progress toward spiritual liberation. It was a day of fasting, to abstain not just from food but from negative words, deeds, and thoughts.

Later that morning, the crowd assembled in and around one of the pilgrim sheds, which had been converted into an auditorium. On the stage, a silver statue of Sai Baba of Shirdi was placed on an urn shaped like a serpent. Sathya Sai Baba walked out to perform a ceremonial bath. First he materialized a statue of Ganesh, Shiva's elephant-headed son, and placed it on the silver statue's head. Then, as the crowd sang *bhajans*, Sai Baba held up a small vase and poured *vibhuti* over the idols. The ash kept flowing, far more than such a vessel could seemingly hold. There seemed to be pearls and precious stones intermixed with it, filling the serpentine urn. Devi felt herself falling into a trance, losing all sense of what was going on around her. When she opened her eyes, the ritual was over and the auditorium was nearly empty.

Shivarathri's miracles had barely begun. At the ashram, the most exciting part of the holiday was the ecstatic all-night vigil that reached its apotheosis when Sai Baba produced lingams, the phallic oval objects that symbolize Shiva. This, more than anything else, was what Devi and thirty thousand others had longed to witness.

By the time evening approached, every inch of space at the ashram was occupied by yearning devotees. Walking around was nearly impossible. All eyes turned toward the Shanti Vedika, the ashram's elevated rotunda, bathed in bright lights, where the night's mysteries would unfold. People camped out for hours to be close to it, but as a foreigner, Devi would have been escorted to a privileged VIP area nearby.

At around 6:00 p.m., Sai Baba took the stage with a group of disciples. He spoke in Telugu about the meaning of the lingam as a symbol of God. He led the crowd in *bhajans*, whose delivery grew faster and more rapturous as the hours went on. Then he began to cough. He'd start to sing again, and then would stop, struggling. He appeared to be in pain. The crowd knew what was happening, since it proceeded this way every year. Over and over, they repeated the last line Baba had uttered, an urgent prayer. His agony seemed to mount until, finally, he held a white towel under his chin and the first lingam came out of his mouth and dropped onto it.

Baba was known to produce lingams made of all sorts of precious materials. This one, egg-shaped and four inches long, was the color of amethyst. The crowd's singing became ecstatic. A second, smaller lingam of the same color emerged from Sai Baba's mouth. He left the stage, and the lingams were placed on a flower-covered tray. The singing continued till dawn.

In the morning, Devi volunteered to help serve the food that was distributed to break the fast. She wondered how the ashram's little kitchen could prepare meals for so many thousands of people and was told that the dishes multiplied at Sai Baba's touch. "Why are you so surprised?" asked one young man. "Didn't Christ feed a multitude with five loaves of bread and two fish?"

Over the following days, Devi was thrilled to find herself pulled into this Christ-like figure's inner circle. Shortly after the Shivarathri festival, Sai Baba was due to travel to Bombay with a group of boys from the ashram school who were going to perform a musical about the life of Krishna. He asked Devi to come along. The caravan stopped for lunch in the village of Hampi, set amid the ruins of an ancient capital and dominated by an ornate, pyramid-shaped Shiva temple. Narayana Kasturi, Sai Baba's official biographer, describes how much fun the guru had showing the boys around: "He caressed them lovingly like a mother and attended to the demands of their curiosity and wonder about the areas through which they passed."

In Bombay, they stayed in a large, old colonial bungalow on the city's outskirts. Sai Baba's fame was spreading, and every morning, thousands of devotees gathered outside to sing *bhajans*, overflowing the lawn and crowding the streets outside. At 9:00 a.m., the avatar would emerge to wander among the throng, blessing household objects, accepting beseeching letters, or simply letting people touch his feet and experience his *darshan*.

The boys performed their play, written by Baba, for an eminent audience that included the governor of Maharashtra, the enormous state that had Bombay (now Mumbai) as its capital. Sai Baba addressed teeming crowds in city stadiums. An elderly man named Ramakrishna Rao, a hero of the independence movement and the onetime governor of Uttar Pradesh, one of India's largest states, stood beside him, interpreting from Telugu into Hindi. Like Vivekananda, Sai Baba spoke of India as a light unto the world: "The greed and selfishness that are infecting this country are tragedies for humanity, for India has the role of guiding and leading mankind to the goal of self-realization."

For Devi, the week in Bombay was like a "fairy tale," each day suffused with whimsical magic. One day, as she sat on the bungalow's veranda, Sai Baba came out followed by a local Bombay politician. He was trying to fit onto his finger a ring that Baba had given him, but it was too tight. Sai Baba took the ring, put it in his palm, and blew on it, and when he handed it back, not only did it fit, but it was now adorned with precious stones. Devi was amazed. "That is nothing," another devotee told her. "I have seen him return sight to a blind man by just blowing into his eyes."

Devi was flying home from Bombay, and on the morning of her departure, Baba lit a temple lamp for her Crusade for Light in Darkness and gave her a silver medallion bearing his image. "Be happy," he told her. Happy didn't begin to describe it.

PART IV

MATAJI

· CHAPTER 15 ·

I N THE EARLY 1970S, Samuel Sandweiss, a San Diego psychiatrist, was growing disenchanted with his field. Outwardly, he was quite successful—in addition to conducting his private practice, he was an assistant clinical professor at the University of California, overseeing psychiatric residents. Yet he was increasingly convinced that psychiatry neglected both the moral and spiritual realms, contributing to a culture of selfishness and hedonism. It overvalued rationality and individualism at the expense of intuition and interconnection.

Sandweiss was intrigued by new currents in psychology that seemed to combine the insights of East and West, particularly the Gestalt therapy of Fritz Perls, which was hugely influential in the more intellectual precincts of the counterculture. Gestalt therapy sought to reveal the ego as a story and a performance instead of an unchanging reality—an idea with parallels to the yogic distinction between the mind and the true self. The aim was to break out of the narratives that imprison us in order to live entirely in the present. It was, in the words of the scholar Jeffrey J. Kripal, "a psychology of pure consciousness, of pristine awareness in the here and now without a why." Some people half-jokingly called it Zen Judaism.

Submitting himself to Gestalt therapy, Sandweiss found it helpful but ultimately unsatisfying; it couldn't ameliorate his deep-seated horror of aging and death. So he decided to look beyond psychology altogether. The therapies he'd been experimenting with, he suspected, approached "yogic or 'spiritual' practices known for thousands of years in the East." Why not go straight to the source?

His search for a yoga and meditation teacher led him, naturally, to Indra Devi, whose Tecate headquarters was only fifty miles away from his home. Crossing the U.S.-Mexico border, he and his wife, Sharon, drove down a narrow dirt road through the foothills until they arrived at Rancho Cuchuma. He was at once taken with the silence and the sunbaked tranquility. "I had the strange feeling of entering another world, removed by more than distance from the hustle of San Diego," he wrote. The two went inside and were immediately struck by a large poster of an Indian man with an afro wearing an orange robe and surrounded by reverent devotees.

Coming down the stairs, Devi charmed the couple at once. Somehow, as she got into her seventies, she seemed to have become only more girlish and effervescent. "I had the impression that she was marvelously open, as if I could actually feel a breeze passing through her body," wrote Sandweiss. As she led them through the house, she sang a *bhajan* to herself.

Soon, scarcely able to contain herself, she started telling them about her swami. Indeed, as she spoke, every topic led back to him. Instead of being annoyed, Sandweiss was intrigued. Devi was no naïve flower child. She'd been all over India and had met some of the country's most renowned holy men. Yet Sai Baba alone had enthralled her. She began to dilate on his miracles—the *vibhuti*, the materializations, the healings. She told Sandweiss that Sai Baba had raised a man from the dead—an elderly American devotee named Walter Cowan, whom Baba was said to have revived after a fatal heart attack in Madras earlier that year.

Sandweiss didn't exactly believe Devi, but he was fascinated by the strength of her conviction. This wasn't an uncommon occurrence. "You see people like Swami Satchidananda and Indra Devi, who have eyes that shine, who radiate so much love that you feel great just being around them, and you start to think, well, maybe they know something, maybe they're right," a Los Angeles yoga student told *Harper's* in 1971. "I've even started to consider enlightenment. The more I think about it, the more irresistible it becomes."

Sandweiss wasn't ready to admit to himself that he was looking for enlightenment, but he grew convinced that Sai Baba had something to teach him. "I felt that observing Baba in person would give me an idea of what might have happened at the time of Christ to propagate those incredible stories," he writes. Devi would soon be taking a group of people to India to meet this modern messiah, something she'd been doing regularly. Sandweiss decided to go along.

By the late 1960s, Devi had become Sai Baba's most important Western evangelist. Five months after her second visit to Puttaparthi, she went back a third time, volunteering as an asana teacher at Sai Baba's boys' school. He regularly oversaw her classes, which delighted her and underlined her importance in the ashram's informal hierarchy. On Krishna Jayanti, a holiday that commemorates Krishna's birth, Sai Baba asked Devi to address the worshippers during the temple celebration. After putting a garland of flowers around Baba's neck and ceremonially touching his feet, she spoke to the assembled thousands, marveling that the miraculous events surrounding Krishna's sojourn on earth were being recapitulated in modern times. "All the miracles which had been performed then, are again being performed now," she said.

How could she help but want to tell the world? Returning to Tecate, she regaled her students, her friends, everyone she met, with stories about Sai Baba. She started lecturing about Sai Baba throughout California, showing a grainy film of the Shivarathri festival. Her husband was skeptical but supportive and even gave her a couple of rooms in his Sunset Boulevard office to start the Sai Baba Foundation, where Los Angeles acolytes could gather to sing *bhajans* and discuss Baba's glory.

She had no trouble finding receptive audiences for her astonishing stories. This was, after all, a uniquely fertile moment for Indian holy men. In 1967 the *New York Times* reported that the Indian consulate was receiving at least twenty calls a week from people seeking yoga lessons or Indian spiritual teachers. Disenchanted with Western religion, great numbers of Americans and Europeans were, like the Theosophists before them, turning east in search of salvation or at least enduring wisdom.

No one symbolized this trend more than the bearded, beatific Maharishi Mahesh Yogi, inventor of Transcendental Meditation. In 1967, the year the Beatles, Mick Jagger, Marianne Faithfull, and others took a course with the Maharishi in Wales, the *New York Times Magazine* declared him "Chief Guru of the Western World." In September, when he flew to Los Angeles, three thousand students showed up to meet his plane.

The expansion of the Maharishi's movement throughout the 1960s mirrored the growth of American yoga. Both first took root among rather square elites and then spread to the counterculture before being reappropriated by the mainstream. The Maharishi's first American supporters were, in the words of Philip Goldberg, "citizens of *Ozzie and Harriet*'s America—clean-shaven dads with neat haircuts and good jobs, and apron-wearing moms who supervised nuclear families in homes equipped with the latest appliances." His Transcendental Meditation, like Devi's yoga, offered itself as a tool for those seeking greater happiness, productivity, and contentment—in other words, those trying to adjust more effectively to the status quo. He was popular with socialites; tobacco heiress Doris Duke put up the money to build his Rishikesh ashram.

As the 1960s progressed, however, the flavor of American romance with Eastern religion changed. The young people increasingly turning toward Indian gurus weren't seeking a calming way to shore up conventional American middle-class life; they were seeking an alternative to it. Hippies—the word had come into circulation in 1965—were influenced by Beats such as Allen Ginsberg, who had wandered the Indian subcontinent in the early 1960s looking for ecstasy, or at least something beyond the "shit and desire" of quotidian existence. Some had tried mushrooms or acid but wanted a more authentic, lasting form of mind expansion—techniques of cosmic bliss, not just health and happiness.

Meanwhile, in 1965, the quota system that had restricted Asian immigration to the United States was abolished, allowing a trickle of Hindu holy men to make their way to the country. That year, A. C. Bhaktivedanta Swami Prabhupata, a Calcutta pharmaceuticals manufacturer turned monk, arrived in New York, where, from a Lower East Side storefront, he taught a form of devotion based on the repetitive, ecstatic chanting of Krishna's name. His followers, who soon became known as Hare Krishnas, would spend hours singing in Tompkins Square Park. When a *New York Times* reporter visited them in the fall of 1966, he found Ginsberg among the celebrants. "It brings a state of ecstasy," Ginsberg said. "For one thing, the syllables force yoga breath control."

Soon Bhaktivedanta expanded westward. Ginsberg wrote with prophetic solemnity, "And a second center for chanting Krishna's Name was thereafter established in San Francisco's Haight-Ashbury at the height of the spiritual crisis and breakthrough renowned in that city, mid-sixties twentieth century." By 1967, Ginsberg and the guru were presiding over a "Mantra-Rock Dance" at the Avalon Ballroom featuring the Grateful Dead and Big Brother and the Holding Company. Though Bhaktivedanta's creed was deeply austere—Hare Krishnas abjured drugs, extramarital sex, meat, and even caffeine—he intuited that he'd find followers among the pleasure-seeking youth. Hippies, he said, "are our best potential. Although they are young, they are already dissatisfied with material life. Frustrated. And not knowing what to do, they turn to drugs. So let them come, and we will show them spiritual activities. Once they engage in Krishna consciousness, all these *anarthas*, unwanted things, will fall away."

A host of lesser-known gurus found American followings as well. In *Life* magazine, Jane Howard described two weeks spent on New York's "Swami Circuit," "a loose network of holy men who in a remarkable sort of brain drain, or spirit drain, have been drifting in from caves and ashrams back in India to fulfill their earthly destiny this time round by setting up institutes and centers all over America." The venues, Howard wrote, "range from slummy storefronts to chic brownstones, but they have one thing in common: none is big enough to handle the swelling crowds who drop by to exercise, chant or meditate and, through these ancient disciplines of mind and body, reach the ultimate goal: bliss." One young woman told the journalist, "all my friends who went to shrinks five years ago are going to swamis now."

Unlike these swamis, whom he often disparaged, Sai Baba never came to the West. He told Devi there were too many gurus in America, "each known by the amount of money he is charging." (Indeed, despite promising her that he'd visit Tecate, he left India only once in his life, on a 1968 trip to Kenya and Uganda, East African countries with large Indian diasporas.) Staying away from the United States and Europe ensured that even as his Indian following grew to eclipse those of other gurus, he'd never be as internationally well known as figures such as the Maharishi Mahesh Yogi. That, however, only increased his appeal to intrepid Western seekers. To encounter Sai Baba, you had to go on an old-fashioned pilgrimage, one that promised not just wisdom, but also miracles. And if you didn't feel like plunging into India on your own, Devi would guide you.

Devi began taking groups of Westerners to India to meet Sai Baba in 1968, and by 1975, nine years after her conversion, she'd made nineteen trips to see him. His followers often referred to her as Mataji, an honorific form of "Mother." For ashram novices, traveling with her was the easiest way to get close to the guru. Baba was famously capricious and would keep some visitors waiting weeks for one of his coveted private audiences. His followers adored his playful unpredictability, seeing in it a divine whimsy characteristic of Indian gods, but for an impatient American with limited time, it was immensely frustrating. Those traveling with Devi, however, could usually be assured of meeting him. Indeed, at both Prasanthi Nilayam and

Brindavan, Sai Baba's summer residence in the Bangalore suburb of Whitefield, everyone with her would be treated like a VIP.

At the start of her first group visit, Baba sent beautiful new saris to the women in her party of thirteen, saying that the garments were easier to wear while sitting on the ground than Western dresses. Then, during the group's audience, he produced for Devi a *jap-mala* (a sort of Indian rosary) made of pearls, which he said she could use to cure others. It was as if he were endowing her with some of his supernatural gifts. "The jap-mala created quite a stir in Prasanthi Nilayam," Devi writes, obviously proud. Everywhere she went, people would ask to see it, then press it reverently to their faces. Some claimed that, afterward, their physical afflictions were lifted.

Sai Baba visited Devi's group every day at their guesthouse, giving them private lectures on his reassuringly ecumenical religious philosophy. They must always avoid sectarianism and fanaticism, he said. All those who revere God, however they describe him, are brothers: "God is only one."

During that trip, the great ophthalmologist M. C. Modi, whose eye surgery clinics gave sight to millions of poor Indians, set up a camp sponsored by Baba in Puttaparthi. Thousands of blind and nearly blind people poured into the ashram, and Modi conducted lightning-fast examinations. Those he could help were laid on a row of assembly-line-style operating tables. He'd move from one to the next, performing surgeries with a flick of his scalpel. As soon as he was finished with patients, volunteers from the ashram would carry them away to recuperate and lay new people in their place. In just a few days the surgeon completed more than five hundred operations. On the last day, when all the patients' bandages had been removed, Baba gave Dr. Modi traditional sarongs to distribute to the men, and he had Devi hand out new saris to the women.

It was exhilarating to be part of such undeniably good works, and Devi was struck by the way Baba remained lighthearted in the midst of it all. One overzealous female volunteer was scandalized by the way the half-blind peasants sat in mixed-sex groups, contrary to ashram policy. When she brought this to Sai Baba's attention, he brushed off the violation. "Doesn't matter, let them," he said, adding with a smile, "They can't see the difference anyway!"

In 1970, when John Lennon and Yoko Ono arrived without warning at Baba's ashram on the eve of his birthday, Devi was given the job of chaperoning them. It didn't strike her as much of an honor— she was so out of touch with pop culture that she kept calling the legendary Beatle "Mr. Lemmon." The couple, in turn, weren't particularly impressed with what they saw. They refused to sit separately in the men's and women's sections of the prayer hall, instead holding hands throughout Baba's talk. Ten years later, in a long joint interview published in *Playboy* two days before Lennon's assassination, Ono described Sai Baba as a showman. "In India you have to be a guru instead of a pop star . . . Guru is the pop star of India, and pop star is the guru here."

Samuel Sandweiss arrived in India with Devi and her party in May 1972, and like many first-time visitors to the country, he found that the heat, the squalor, and the surging masses of people made him wish he could turn around and go home. Baba had organized a school of spirituality for Indian college students at Brindavan, and Devi had arranged for Sandweiss to sit in on the classes, which would be given by guest lecturers, and to attend the guru's evening discourses.

His first letters home to his wife, included in a book he later wrote, are full of impatience, frustration, and doubt. The school's emphasis on strict sexual morality was jarring. When one of the teachers informed the students that negative thoughts were the same as negative deeds, it offended Sandweiss's psychiatric sensibility. He found Sai Baba fascinating—"He has a high smooth voice, bright eyes and the quickness of a cat," he wrote. "He often acts with childlike innocence but can change in a wink to a commanding, powerful figure." But a God? Sandweiss was far from convinced.

Still, he longed to be. In his book, he admits that he'd been nurturing fantasies of returning to America as a modern-day apostle, "a great bringer of the word of God . . . marched down the streets of the USA on shoulders of admirers." He felt desperate to see a miracle. For all his claims to skepticism, his dreams for a huge and meaningful life depended on Sai Baba being who he said he was.

Meanwhile, the more he listened to Baba, the less attached he felt to the liberal Western convictions he'd arrived with. "I now wonder why I have such faith in my value system, for this system is the reflection of a culture which isn't doing very well," he wrote to his wife a week after arriving. "Half the marriages in Southern California now end in divorce; people are raping the land, polluting the air and killing each other, and there seems little regard for love or for God." With self-indulgence so utterly unsatisfying, perhaps he shouldn't be so quick to reject the value of discipline, the peace to be found in aligning one's life with eternal verities. "Baba gives people the strength to believe in these forgotten attitudes," he wrote.

Two days later he saw his first miracle: Baba materialized a religious medallion and placed it around a professor's neck. "Amazing! Unbelievable! Unthinkable!" Sandweiss writes. He was becoming convinced that the stories in the Bible were not allegories but fact. "The divine *does* become manifest in order to teach," he writes. "God *does* appear on earth. There are forces in the universe, powers of being, that we cannot even imagine."

Sandweiss eventually became a leader in the Sai Baba movement, and in 1975 he published his influential book *The Holy Man . . . and the Psychiatrist*, a hit in New Age bookstores. He even converted one of his psychiatric residents. "For two years we met and he told me stories of this man of miracles," writes psychiatrist Dennis Gersten. "The miracle stories shook my very foundation of reality." Gersten eventually accompanied Sandweiss to meet the guru in India, after which he concluded, "There is no miracle known to humankind that Sai Baba has not performed."

That year, Devi published her own book, *Sai Baba and Sai Yoga*, which attempted to marry asana practice to Sai Baba devotion. The short volume is divided in half: first comes a hagiographic account of her miraculous encounters with the guru, and then instructions for assuming yoga poses, coupled with messages of spiritual uplift and suggestions for meditation. Sai Yoga, writes Devi, depended on learning the postures so well that one no longer needed to think about the position of the body while practicing them and could instead turn the mind toward the divine. As a *Yoga Journal* writer described Sai Yoga, "The main pose of each class includes an invocation, so that the fulcrum of each practice involves a meditation in the form of an ecumenical prayer."

From time to time, Sai Baba would suddenly start criticizing or ignoring a previously favored disciple. In his book *Lord of the Air*, Tal Brooke, an edgy young ex-acidhead, longhaired and bearded, whom Sai Baba nicknamed "Rowdie," describes the first time it happened to him. It was during a meeting of the leadership of Sai Baba's Indian organizations, a group that included thousands, many of them members of the country's political and business elite. Devi was speaking, and Baba asked Brooke to address the audience after her.

During her talk, Devi repeated one of her favorite stories, about driving on a crowded Los Angeles six-lane freeway when one of her front tires blew out. As the car careened out of control and oncoming Mack trucks threatened to crush her, she screamed, "Sai Ram!" and made it safely to the grassy median. Baba smiled at her as she left the stage. Then it was Brooke's turn.

His talk attempted to synthesize Sai Baba's message with Christianity: "It was Truth that turned the world upside down after Christ had come, and it will be the same Spirit of Truth at work in this age . . . The wickedness of the Roman empire is here again today. This time it is the Kali Yuga mentioned in the Agni Purana—that Bible calls it 'the Great Tribulation.'"

There was nothing particularly unusual in this sort of conflation. Sai Baba had always subsumed the world's faiths into his own message, and in fact, the ashram's logo was a picture of a lotus with the symbols of the world's major religions—a Christian cross, an Islamic star and crescent, a Hindu Om, a Buddhist wheel, a Zoroastrian fire sign—in its petals. (In some versions, there's also a Jewish Star of David.) He gave Christmas discourses and frequently spoke of Jesus, especially with his Western devotees. "Call me by any name—Krishna, Allah, Christ," he'd said in 1968.

When Brooke was finished, Devi stepped across the red carpet dividing the hall's men's section from the women's section—a boundary she often flouted, with singular impunity—and threw her arms around him. In his book, Brooke renders her accent as vaguely Transylvanian, quoting her as saying, "Thatt vas turrific."

When he saw Baba, however, the guru barely acknowledged him. "Too long," he grumbled. "Too fast speaking. Words too complicated. American accent not understanding. Not enough surrender, sir."

Brooke protested that his accent hadn't changed and that everyone had understood his previous speeches. "Indra Devi just now tell me that she not understand," Baba replied.

Had Devi really been that two-faced? Brooke found her and asked if she'd spoken to Baba after his speech. She insisted that she hadn't.

He told her what Baba had said. "He must be testing you," she said. "I've been tested many times. Don't let it get your goat. He only does that to his most favored disciples."

That didn't make it any easier when Baba turned on her. In 1974 Devi was part of Sai Baba's entourage during a trip to Sanduru, a mining town a hundred fifty miles away from Puttaparthi, where he was to lay the foundation stone for a new plant, inaugurate a public park, and be received by the local maharaja. On the way back, she writes vaguely, he accused her "of things I had neither said nor done." She tried to talk to him when they returned to the ashram, but he was avoiding her. Hurt, she decided to go home early.

As soon as she reached California, she went to see her mother. Then in her nineties and living in a nursing home, Sasha hated her daughter's constant traveling. When Devi arrived at her side, it quickly became clear that Sasha didn't have much longer to live. Devi stayed with her mother overnight, and according to *Sai Baba and Sai Yoga*, Sasha died early the next morning. Later, when Devi had drifted away from her guru, she stopped telling this story, so perhaps the timing wasn't quite so precise. For the moment, though, Devi's faith in Sai Baba was renewed. He had sent her to be with her mother when she was most needed.

Devi had loved Sasha more than anyone on earth. She was, she writes, "my friend and companion throughout every adventure of my life." Still, protected by the detachment she'd spent a lifetime cultivating, she did not give herself over to grief or let herself dwell on death. Her childhood horror of coffins had never dissipated—instead, it had expanded to include hearses and everything associated with burial. Thus, instead of giving her a Russian Orthodox funeral, she had her mother cremated and scattered her ashes into the Pacific Ocean. As she said her last good-byes, she didn't cry, believing that her mother had simply moved on to another plane.

This ability to avoid suffering, to hold part of herself aloof from even the most searing losses, was something she'd been working toward since she first discovered yoga. From the Bhagavad Gita, she writes, she'd learned the paramount importance of two "fundamental virtues," love and nonattachment. Attachment turned love into a prison, she believed, but without love, nonattachment was cold and sterile. Through yoga, she was convinced it was possible to love without ever experiencing the anguish of loss or the constriction of dependency. That doesn't mean, however, that those close to her were able to do the same.

When Devi first started going back and forth to India, Dr. Knauer stayed behind in California. He didn't like her constant traveling any more than Sasha had, but he knew better than to try to stop her. Until he was in his late seventies, his work continued to fill up most of his time, though at some point—precisely when is unclear—authorities cracked down on his unorthodox cancer cures. Losing his license, he "spirited away to his home across the Mexican border carloads of his precious remedies," in the words of Nancy Poer, a close friend and patient, and set up a practice in Tecate. Devoted patients from California would drive over the border for his ministrations.

Often when Devi returned from one of her innumerable trips, he'd meet her at the airport with flowers. In Tecate, they sometimes worked in tandem—his patients would take classes with her, and he'd treat her students. At any one time, the place would be full of earnest aspiring yoga teachers, ailing minor aristocrats, and scruffy hippies whom Devi was determined to clean up. Drug addicts came to detox with Dr. Knauer's help and mixed with the socialites popping over from Rancho La Puerta.

Devi grew especially close to one of her students, a beautiful dark-haired woman named Rosita. She stayed on as Devi's assistant, helping to teach classes and handling the administration of the school. Often Devi referred to Rosita as her adopted daughter.

There was a schedule at the ranch, but it wasn't rigidly enforced. Time and again, Devi would spontaneously propose various health regimens. "Who wants to do a watermelon fast?" one of her yoga students, Bettina Biggart, recalled her asking. Everyone would be put to work. "She always had a group of people at her beck and call," said Biggart. "Darling, you do this, you do that."

When Biggart first went to Rancho Cuchuma, she was a yoga teacher in her thirties who had studied with B. K. S. Iyengar. Arriving for a one-month teacher-training course, she was assigned a room with an older German lady who was being treated by Dr. Knauer. The two women immediately bonded, and when Devi swanned in and saw them talking, she said to Biggart, "Darling, she's sick. You just give her a coffee enema."

"Mataji," Biggart replied, "I don't know how to give enemas."

Having none of it, Devi fetched the enema bag and gave her pupil a quick explanation. "Here's this stranger that I've been asked to give an enema," said Biggart. "Somehow I did it, and the next day she was well enough to come to the class."

Under Devi's guidance, both women became Sai Baba devotees.

Dr. Knauer had his first stroke one Christmas Eve in Los Angeles, when he and Devi were taking care of last-minute errands before heading to Tecate for the holiday. Devi knew something was wrong when her husband, a usually punctilious driver, sailed through several red lights without noticing. She looked at him and saw that his face was contorted. Soon he started losing his vision, and half his body became paralyzed.

After a while he started to recover and was able to resume his work in Mexico. Hoping Sai Baba could fully cure him, Devi convinced her husband to accompany her to Puttaparthi, renting a house for them on the ashram's outskirts. It was a punishing journey even for a young, healthy person and was hard on the aging doctor, an austere, orderly man who had never liked the dirt and chaos of India. There, Sai Baba materialized thirty-three pills, which he said were to be taken daily. When Knauer got worse, the guru said it was his karma at work and must be accepted.

In 1980 Knauer suffered another stroke, one that would leave him needing a full-time caregiver. Devi had no intention of stepping into this role; her freedom was too important to her, her antipathy to quotidian domestic obligations too deep. Knauer went to stay with Nancy Poer and her husband, Gordon. "There gathered around him a large community of friends, providing care, special food, and funds," Poer writes. "Soon the house filled with flowers, old friends, children who played the harp and flute, and dozens of souls to meet and support him." With their solicitude, he began to improve, and was able to celebrate his eighty-sixth birthday at a gala party. "One felt that those present represented a microcosm of his world-flung practice . . . various races and nationalities, the very old, the famous, tanned teenagers and babes in arms," writes Poer.

Yet Devi, who loved her husband even if she wouldn't make many sacrifices for him, wanted Knauer with her. Rosita, her assistant, had married one of Dr. Knauer's protégés and was spending less and less time in Tecate. Both strong, demanding personalities, Devi and Rosita's husband found themselves in a power struggle for Rosita's attention. As Devi tells the story, Rosita, uncomfortable in the middle, eventually told Devi she couldn't work with her anymore. Devi understood—she knew she could be a prima donna—and wished her well. Without Rosita, though, she couldn't maintain both her school and her peripatetic life. She decided to take Dr. Knauer and move to India, using their savings to buy a house in Whitefield, where they could live out their lives in the shadow of the avatar.

As it happened, the avatar was not particularly pleased about this. Devi was far more useful to Sai Baba in the Americas than in India, and he wanted her to stay put. Even the will of God, however, was no match for her restlessness.

Knauer's friends were understandably horrified. Almost everyone he loved was in California; there was nothing for him in India except his wife, who could scarcely be counted on to stay by his side. Years later, when a friend and former patient penned an obituary for Knauer in an Anthroposophical Society newsletter, the anger at Devi was still raw. "For some reason known only to the angel of destiny, Sigfrid Knauer was to finish his long life in the East," wrote Barbara Betteridge. There, she continued, "he was further estranged from all he had known. Children and grandchildren were far away. Blind, he could not even read his beloved Rudolf Steiner, and there was often no one to speak or read to him in any of the four languages he had lived by."

Devi, though, was determined, and heedless of her husband's needs. Initially she enlisted a young man named Paul O'Brien to help her husband make the journey. At the time, O'Brien was a seeker who yearned to undertake a great global pilgrimage, visiting sacred sites the world over. He wanted to meet a truly enlightened being—and he hoped that getting out of the country would help him escape his cocaine habit. In preparation for his travels, he signed up for a ten-day meditation course at a California ashram. At the end of it, Devi came to lecture. Her talk, aptly, was about the relationship between love and nonattachment.

"She was so sweet throughout, and she just enchanted everybody," O'Brien told me. At the end of her speech, she announced that she was looking for two men to travel with her husband in exchange for airfare and room and board when they arrived. It seemed like a perfect opportunity, and O'Brien wrote her an impassioned letter about why she should choose him. Impressed, she told him to get ready to leave. When he called back, though, he was told he was no longer needed. Apparently, Devi had found others, perhaps with medical experience, to take care of Knauer. O'Brien didn't try to hide his surprise and disappointment, but Devi told him, "We have something else for you. I want you to help me write my autobiography."

It was a project Devi had long been planning. She routinely saved the biographical sketches people wrote to introduce her at various events, and made scattered notes and time lines that she intended, someday, to turn into a book. Thus O'Brien ended up in India as Devi's secretary and amanuensis, though in the end she was too restive to devote any real time to the project. She told him stories, and he wrote them down, but he couldn't get her to work systematically. They traveled around the country constantly—Devi was always being invited to spiritual festivals. Sometimes, she would go on the road with Baba. "I could never get her to sit still," O'Brien said. She might have preached the necessity of stilling the mind, but she'd never been much interested in keeping her own ricocheting enthusiasms in check. What she called detachment occasionally looked more like whirling escapism. Knauer, meanwhile, was stranded in Whitefield in the care of hired aides.

In her restlessness, Devi had embarked on a new project: building schools for local street kids with money raised through her revived Crusade for Light organization. As one of her foundation fundraising letters somewhat cringingly put it, "One day she went out into the street and literally called out, 'who wants to go to school?' In an instant she was surrounded by eager, hungry little faces." She found a room in the village of Sorahunase, four miles away from her home in Whitefield, and hired an instructor to teach Hindi, English, and handicrafts—she herself would teach yoga and *bhajans*. Called Sai Kiran, the school was inaugurated with a speech by Narayana Kasturi, Sai Baba's biographer and a major figure in the Sai organization.

At around the same time, Devi wrote that she came across a group of small children whose mothers left them in a dark garage while they went to work in a factory nearby; they were, in the words of the fund-raising letter, "all huddled together like a basket of tiny kittens." For them, Devi opened a nursery. She also began providing meals and yoga lessons for some of the street kids in her neighborhood.

Bettina Biggart helped her raise money for this work, from Sai Baba devotees in the United States. People were generous, Biggart said, "because [the money] went straight to take care of the kids. She's not paying any salaries, she cleaned these kids up, these kids were getting an education." Whenever Devi visited California, she'd solicit funds herself. "When she turned on the charm, it was a sight to behold," said Biggart, who recalled one Hollywood producer writing a check for twenty-five thousand dollars.

Devi was doing useful work, but she found the small scale of it unsatisfying. She started to think bigger. A 1980 fund-raising let-ter said that Sai Kiran was "only the first phase of a model village project" that would serve "as a host community, when living quar-ters are built, for others from identical villages to learn to practice the principles of living by mutual support systems." This idea was abandoned, however, and instead Devi decided to build a pyramid-shaped temple that could serve as a school, a yoga center, and a place for spiritual lectures. When the Hollywood producer who'd given her twenty-five thousand dollars heard that that was where it was going, he was livid. Biggart was embarrassed on Devi's behalf, but Devi, as always, was blithely unapologetic.

"That's the way she was with money," said Biggart, exasperated and affectionate. Devi never set out to con anyone. It's just that her devotion to nonattachment sometimes extended to her own prom-ises, as well as her own cash. At some point she'd started carrying thousands of dollars at a time in her purse, which she was always losing. "Mataji, why are you doing that?" asked Biggart, alarmed by the large sums Devi kept on hand. "Well, you never know, darling," Devi replied. In someone else, this might have looked like senility or a distrust of banks rooted in her tumultuous history. In Devi, though, such defiant impracticality was part of her insouciant cha-risma, at least to those who loved her.

Meanwhile, in Whitefield, Knauer was suffering horribly. He told his wife he couldn't imagine what he had done in a previous life to deserve such a miserable end. She was saddened by his decline, but she refused to let it dominate her life. "It wasn't like she was ever going to be sitting at somebody's bedside for very long," said O'Brien. "She was peripatetic, adventurous, rambunctious and high energy. There's no way she's going to be domesticated."

Devi's callousness was striking, particularly in one who held herself out as a spiritual teacher. At Sai Baba's ashram, people gossiped about the way she treated Knauer. Baba himself was unhappy. "One time Baba said, 'Where is she running off to; why isn't she taking care of her husband?'" said Biggart. "A lot of us would go and spend time with him. The man was so brilliant. It was pretty hard on such a brilliant man. He didn't have a chance to do anything but read."

Devi never tried to defend herself. In her memoirs, she acknowledges that she was constantly on the road and that she spent little time with her husband. "But I never claimed to be something I wasn't, and those who know me know that I'm not a conventional woman, and that I practice what I call 'Love and Detachment,'" she writes.

She never stopped believing that personal spiritual development came before relationships. In the Hindu spiritual culture she lionized, the householder who abandons everything, family included, to become a wandering ascetic is revered. Devi was no ascetic, but she found sanction in that tradition for her own roaming. Years later, speaking of married couples to Roberto Díaz Herrera, a Panamanian colonel who idolized her, she put it this way: "I do not understand how they can let the other person, whoever they may be, stop their mission in life. How will you explain that to God? Imagine: 'God, my wife did not let me grow!' or 'I had a bad husband!'"

Critics of the Western embrace of Eastern religion have often feared that it would nurture attitudes such as this one. If it's possible to be at once nonattached and deeply emotionally enmeshed with family and friends, few have figured out how. Nor are many Americans or Europeans—Devi very much included—truly interested in the systematic dissolution of the ego that is a goal of Hindu and Buddhist disciplines. Instead, in a strange sort of inversion, New Age movements have often used Eastern spiritual techniques to strengthen individualism.

In 1977, Harvey Cox, a left-wing Christian theologian with a serious Buddhist meditation practice, decried what he viewed as the moral hazard inherent in the Western appropriation of Eastern philosophies. "What comes out looks much like irresponsibility with a spiritual cover, a metaphysical license to avoid risky, demanding relationships, a mystical permit to skip from one person, bed, cause or program to another without ever taking the plunge," he writes. Devi's treatment of her husband is surely the sort of thing Cox is talking about.

Yet it also seems that Devi's practice of detachment served her, if not those around her, quite well. Knauer's agonizing decline appeared to cause her little suffering, at least consciously. (Anyone with a psychoanalytic bent will likely see her frenzied activity during these years as an escape mechanism.) Her detachment was so well developed that it extended to faith itself. It meant that, unlike many of those caught up in the Eastern cults of the 1960s and '70s, she would emerge unscathed when things started to fall apart.

WHEN INDRA DEVI met the Swedish Sai Baba devotee Conny Larsson at the beginning of 1981, he was the talk of both Whitefield and Puttaparthi. Several months earlier, while at home in Sweden, he shattered his knee in an accident with a horse, and he was still on crutches when he traveled to Prasanthi Nilayam. During a Christmas *darshan*, Sai Baba called Larsson to the front of the *mandir*, or temple, and, before tens of thousands of people, ordered him to throw his crutches aside and walk. Somehow he did it, electrifying Sai Baba's flock. Larsson later insisted that he'd already been on the mend, but at the time, he couldn't admit this to himself, let alone anyone else.

"I was caught in his net and also felt the pressure from the thousands of believers who witnessed the spectacle," he writes. "We were only too willing to believe, and who was I to diminish Sai Baba, my God?" Wherever he walked in the ashram after that, Larsson seemed an embodiment of Baba's astonishing healing powers. People tried to kiss his hands and feet. Soon, the attention at Puttaparthi grew overwhelming, and he decided to go north to Whitefield, where the cultic energy was usually a bit less intense.

There, early in the New Year, Devi approached him in the ashram canteen. She was famous in Sai Baba circles, and though they had never met before, he was immediately drawn to her—the small, white-haired woman appeared radiant, even saintly. As soon as they started talking, he sensed she wasn't really interested in the putative miracle. Instead, she asked him questions that made him uneasy. "She somehow talked to me in a very peculiar way," he said. "She was very friendly, very gentle, the most lovely person I ever had met around Sai Baba, but I didn't sense her as a follower. I sensed her as someone who was on her way out."

Larsson, a former actor who'd been a child star in Sweden, was well known as one of Sai Baba's favorites. The guru always had a few, most of them young men, though Larsson was thirty-two. Sometimes, like Tal Brooke, these favorites would be entrusted to lead *bhajans* or to speak on festival days. They were called in for private interviews more than anyone else. Devi wanted to know what happened during these audiences. Why was Larsson invited so often? Did he go with other people or alone? How did he feel about his relationship with Baba? "She kept on going around in circles, to get some small pieces out," Larsson said.

Over two conversations, in response to her patient probing, he began to tell her how Sai Baba was raising his kundalini energy, which he did by rubbing oil on his penis and massaging his testicles. At this, says Larsson, Devi's soft smile disappeared and her face went gray. "As soon as I saw that reaction, I withdrew a little bit, because I felt ashamed," Larsson said. "She showed me a mirror, her face became a mirror, so I could see that there was something wrong." He didn't reveal everything—that Sai Baba "sucked my cock, he took my sperm and so on," as Larsson said later—but he must have revealed enough to confirm Devi's growing suspicion.

For Larsson, the doubt Devi planted in his mind wouldn't fully flower for many more years. "That was in fact the triggering point that made me think that something was awkward here," he says. "And then of course I later denied that, and since she was away and I never saw her, I forgot about it." Larsson's unease lay dormant until six people were killed in Sai Baba's apartment in 1993, after which he began asking questions and finally turned on the man he'd once seen as God on earth. By then, though, Devi was long gone.

When she met Larsson, Devi had known about the rumors for years. In 1976, Tal Brooke published a febrile, apocalyptic memoir, *Lord of the Air*—later republished as *Avatar of Night*—in which he reveals that Sai Baba molested him and several other devotees, pulling down their flies and masturbating them during private interviews. At first, Brooke writes, he convinced himself that Baba was administering some sort of tantric purification or simply testing Brooke's allegiance. Eventually, however, he came to believe that the guru was deeply evil. Describing one of the last times he saw Baba, Brooke writes that it "felt as though the spirit that inhabited the bright-robed body was so putrid, so foul, so horrifying that if the crowds could just see it for a second denuded, they would scream and run in terror."

Brooke, however, was easy for Baba's followers to dismiss, and not just because of his book's acid purple prose. *Lord of the Air* culminates in Brooke's conversion to evangelical Christianity. It treats Baba not as a fraud, but as the Antichrist. "A sovereign hand and a restraining power seemed to gently cloak me from Baba's venomous crossfire," Brooke writes of his final confrontation with his onetime guru. "I got a very real feeling that an ancient battle was going on about me that I was only dimly aware of, a great controversy between the creature in red and an unnamable infinitely vaster might." Other Christians might have thrilled to Brooke's story of spiritual warfare on the Indian subcontinent, but if you didn't share his faith, you could write him off as an angry fanatic.

Yet other stories kept bubbling up. Indeed, they were only half-secret, since many in Baba's inner circle accepted what he did, seeing it, as Brooke had at first, as either a sacrament or a test. After all, the Judeo-Christian God had commanded Abraham to kill his son to prove his devotion. Was it really so inexplicable for the avatar to demand that his followers demonstrate a willingness to violate their own cherished taboos? When Larsson told another Swedish devotee (a woman who later became his girlfriend) what Sai Baba was doing during their private audiences, he says she didn't seem surprised. "She explained that this act by Baba was of a sacred nature, and only those who were specially chosen were vouchsafed it," he wrote.

Devi never said a word about any of this publicly, but she later told one of her closest friends that she knew what was happening. The realization can't have been easy—she was in her eighties, with no family except her slowly dying husband and nowhere else in the world to go. She had no desire for an ugly public confrontation. Besides, though Devi was disturbed when she learned of Baba's sexual proclivities, she retained faith in his powers.

This was not unusual. Years later, when the advent of the Internet unleashed a flood of stories from devotees coerced into sex with Sai Baba, some when they were young boys, many of his followers declared him beyond ordinary human categories of good and evil, purity and sin.

On the website "Sai Baba—A Clear View," an American devotee calling himself Ram Das Awle writes of struggling with doubts but eventually concluding that Sai Baba was engaged in rarified tantric practices designed to free his followers from sexual karma accumulated over several lifetimes. "Many souls on this planet have had the *karmic* thorn of lust deeply embedded in their hearts, due to repeated misuse of sexual energy in the human realm, thus creating a painful obstacle to their happiness and spiritual evolution," Awle writes. "As an incarnation of God, Baba will know just how to most efficiently remove those thorns, which otherwise could burn and fester in those souls for eons. *Sometimes the best way to remove a thorn is by using a similar thorn to dig it out; then both can be thrown away*" (boldface and italics are Awle's).

Awle even explains away Baba's sexual encounters with children: "[I]t's important to understand that when Baba looks at a person He doesn't just see a human being of a particular age and gender. He sees the soul, an ancient spark of the infinite Divine flame—along with all the accumulated karma and mental tendencies that form that soul's bondage." Further, Awle argues, the ability to accept the seemingly unacceptable was the mark of a true devotee. "*[W]hen He acts in such a way that a doubt is created in our mind about Him . . .* **He is only reflecting the doubt that was already latent within our mind, bringing it to the surface so it can be faced directly.**"

In 2004, BBC News aired an exposé about Sai Baba, *The Secret Swami*. In it, Isaac Tigrett, a cofounder of the Hard Rock Cafe and one of Baba's most well-known followers, says that he believes the rumors about Sai Baba having sex with adolescent boys are probably true, but that they haven't compromised his faith. "He could go out and murder someone tomorrow, as I said, it's not going to change my evolution," says Tigrett.

Devi would never have gone this far; she was much too independent. Yet even when she learned the truth about Baba, she remained silent. Later, she would tell a close friend named Piero that she didn't want to destroy the hope Baba's followers felt. Perhaps she wasn't ready to let go of her own hope, either—or of her place in Baba's organization, the center of her identity, the reason she'd dragged her still-suffering husband away from his home. So she kept quiet about her realization and appeared as ardent as ever in her worship. She continued to travel on Sai Baba's behalf, and wherever she went she hung his picture in her room, along with photos of her mother and Nehru. Yet she was pulling away, looking outside his orbit for another shot at salvation.

Around this time, Devi received a letter from Paul O'Brien, who'd been thrown out of India for overstaying his visa. He'd gone to Sri Lanka to get a new one, and there he discovered a bearded young holy man, Swami Premananda, who claimed to be the reincarnation of Vivekananda. As Premananda well knew, Sai Baba once predicted that Vivekananda would be reborn in Sri Lanka, and the enterprising swami went out of his way to present himself as the embodiment of that prophecy. He often wore a Vivekananda-style turban and demonstrated his divinity with Sai Baba–style materializations and magic tricks.

Premananda's main ashram in Matale, a town in the center of Sri Lanka, was humble. He had only a few thousand followers, a tiny fraction of Sai Baba's, but like Sai Baba, he had a powerful, playful charisma. "He was totally illiterate—he was illiterate in his own language—and yet he had the most magnetic personality of anybody I'd ever met," says O'Brien. "He was so instantly attractive in this weird, Scorpionic sort of way. He was just delightful. He was childlike. He would just laugh, and he was so happy, and yet he had this power—he had this ability to assert authority anytime he wanted."

O'Brien describes once sitting shotgun in a van full of Premananda's followers while the guru drove them to a religious festival. He had no driver's license and careened around wildly, passing cows on the road so closely that a swishing tail hit O'Brien through the open window. Grinning at his terrified passenger, Premananda said, "Swami can drive and materialize at the same time!" With that, he waved his left hand and then handed O'Brien a wad of paste made with the red *kumkum* powder used by Hindus for religious markings. O'Brien looked at him and said, "Swami, that's great. If the police stop you, you can materialize a driving license!" Premananda gave him a big smile and replied, "Nooooo problem!"

O'Brien wasn't completely sure about Premananda's divinity, but he thought Devi should meet him. Besides, he missed her terribly. So he wrote to her, telling her that Vivekananda had returned and was living in Matale. To his delight, she arrived a few days later.

Just as O'Brien thought, she was immediately taken with Premananda, and the guru was gratified to be visited by the woman who'd done so much to make Sai Baba internationally famous. Speaking through an interpreter, he told her that they'd been connected in their previous lives and that their meeting was predestined. "Now she's like his new best friend, he's leveraging her to legitimize himself," says O'Brien.

The next day, they traveled north to the second of Premananda's three ashrams, located in the town of Puliyankulam, in the heart of Sri Lanka's Tamil country. Surrounded by lush green jungle, Devi adored the ashram's atmosphere of "love, devotion and peace." It was a Spartan place, but to Devi, that only added to its charm—she praised the swami's "utter disregard for money, comforts and possessions."

There might have been a subtle rebuke to Sai Baba in these words. As Devi well knew by this point, the guru's rejection of donations was only a pretense. Once in the fold, believers who had funds were encouraged to wire money to a bank in Andhra Pradesh. One of the lesser revelations of Brooke's *Lord of the Air* is that Devi herself gave Sai Baba several hundred thousand rupees, or tens of thousands of dollars. Others donated much more. Tigrett—who made "Love All, Serve All," a Sai Baba saying, the slogan of his Hard Rock Cafes—gave tens of millions of dollars. Much of that money was used for charitable works—Tigrett's money funded the building of a three-hundred-bed hospital in Puttaparthi—but the guru also traveled by Rolls-Royce and lived in veritable palaces.

Premananda, by contrast, slept on a board resting on bricks in a tiny room behind the ashram kitchen.

From Puliyankulam they traveled to the provincial capital of Jaffna, where Premananda had Devi introduce him before one of his public discourses. Ardent devotees welcomed him with garlands of flowers, some of which he bestowed on Devi. When it was time for her to leave for her return trip to India, he materialized a watch for her—she had recently lost hers—and asked her to come back for his thirty-first birthday, on November 17, only ten days away. This would be difficult, because Sai Baba's birthday was on November 23, and there were huge festivities in the works at his ashrams. Yet Premananda was so sweet she couldn't resist.

So a week and a half later she was back. Amid the celebrations, Premananda begged her advice. Should he continue with his humble ashram life or take his Sai Baba–like message to the world, working to awaken people's spiritual energies, to urge them onto the path of love and devotion? Devi told him that the choice was already being made for him—after all, a newspaper had just called him "Sri Lanka's Sai Baba." When one of the devotees at his birthday celebration invited him to visit the Philippines, it seemed to confirm her wisdom.

"Mataji, you must come with me," Premananda pleaded. She had responsibilities in India (including her husband, whose condition was worsening by the day), but again, she couldn't turn him down. Besides, she was readying herself to break with Sai Baba, and she must have known that taking up with Premananda would force the issue. In January 1983 she met the latter in Manila.

Their first day there, he surprised her by shaving off his beard, which she had always hated. Without it, he looked uncannily like a young Sai Baba—he even had the same pouf of wiry hair. Also, like Sai Baba, he was ecumenical—when a Filipino reporter came to interview him, he materialized a crucifix for her.

Their days were filled with receptions, interviews, and lectures, and wherever they went, enthusiastic crowds surrounded them. "Perhaps it is the country's spiritual psyche which has also drawn quite a lot of attention to our faith healers, mystics and other supernatural phenomena, but Swami Premananda felt at 'home' almost immediately here," reported one Manila newspaper.

Devi was embraced as well, staying behind after Premananda left so she could conduct a three-day yoga seminar. She met the Reverend Alex Orbito, a world-renowned practitioner of so-called psychic surgery. In her book *Going Within*, Shirley MacLaine describes how Orbito reached through her skin to heal her: "There was a great deal of sloshing as blood and guts were rocked from side to side . . . He extracted more 'negative stress clots' and soon withdrew first his right hand, then his left." He "operated" on Devi's eye—her eyesight had started to decline, and she was too vain to wear glasses—and the results left her amazed. Orbito was left with a bit of blood on his fingers, she wrote in a letter to friends, but she'd felt no pain at all.

It was all tremendous fun, until she returned to Whitefield. There, she found herself frozen out. To her friends within the Sai Baba movement, it was clear what had happened: she had let her ego run wild, and the master was putting her in her place. "She had to realize even with her exalted position, there were limits, and she didn't recognize the limits," says Biggart. Everyone in Sai Baba's orbit knew he tested people. "These people that are well known and have had a lot of grace from him, he takes them down a peg or two," Biggart says.

Yet rather than waiting and reflecting when her guru stopped paying attention to her, Devi had run off to Premananda. Then, even worse, she'd started talking about her new guru among Sai Baba's followers. "That was the biggest mistake in the world," says Biggart. "I said, 'Mataji, you can't go to the ashram and sit there in the first row and pass around pictures of Premananda.' She said, 'Oh, but darling, he's Baba's devotee!'"

Soon, ashram authorities gave Devi an ultimatum: either swear off Premananda or be banished from Sai Baba's community. With her faith in Baba already attenuated, there was no way she was going to compromise her liberty, though after all he'd meant to her and all she'd done to proselytize for him, it was a painful moment. In her memoir, she says nothing about the sex scandals, framing her break with him as yet another example of her detachment. "I try not to be subject to anything, because I like my freedom," she wrote.

Thus in 1983 she ended her ties with Sai Baba's organization and began making plans to move to Sri Lanka. Premananda was remodeling a large hilltop home to serve as a meditation center, and he suggested that Devi buy the neighboring estate and re-create her yoga school there. She found a nursing home for her husband in Matale, moving him even farther away from anything familiar, and she rented a house across the street.

Then came the Black July riots. There had long been simmering tension and occasional bursts of violence between Sri Lanka's minority Tamils, most of them Hindus like Premananda, and its Sinhalese majority, most of whom are Buddhist. The riots during the summer of 1983, however, marked the outbreak of a full-scale civil war. It began when the Tamil Tigers, a group of guerrilla secessionists, ambushed a Sri Lankan military patrol, killing fifteen soldiers. Vicious anti-Tamil pogroms broke out in response. Hundreds if not thousands of Tamils were murdered—estimates vary widely—and

Tamil homes and businesses were destroyed. Hundreds of thousands of Tamils soon fled the country.

Among them was Premananda, whose meditation center was left in ruins. Along with some of his followers, he resettled in the South Indian state of Tamil Nadu, where he would eventually construct a new ashram.

This left Devi with little reason to stay in the increasingly unstable Sri Lanka. She could spend only so much time by the side of her suffering, debilitated husband. Whenever she asked him what he was doing, he responded, "dying," which she chose to interpret as a sign of his bone-dry sense of humor. Healthy and restless at eighty-four, she was far from done living. Devi's refusal to take care of the people she loved demonstrated the dark side of yoga philosophy—or yoga philosophy as refracted through Western individualism—but her vitality was a testament to yoga's invigorating power. She was ready for new exploits, fresh journeys.

Luckily, an Argentinean rock star had just invited her to Buenos Aires.

B<small>Y THE TIME</small> Piero De Benedictis returned to Buenos Aires in 1981, he had grown weary of the fiery politics that had driven him into exile.

Born in Italy but raised in Argentina, Piero had been a famous balladeer, known throughout Latin America by his first name, like Madonna or Cher. In the early 1970s he became involved with the left wing of the movement calling for the return of populist president Juan Perón, who had been deposed by a military coup in 1955. His music grew increasingly militant—he sang stirring calls for a people's liberation ("Para el pueblo lo que es del pueblo") and excoriations of military involvement in Argentinean politics ("Que se vayan ellos").

After the 1976 military coup that marked the escalation of Argentina's Dirty War, songs such as these could get a person killed. The government's junta kidnapped and murdered as many as thirty thousand left-wing activists and alleged sympathizers, including students and journalists. Censorship was both ubiquitous and capricious. Wrote one scholar: "There were words whose use would be punished, but it was never made known which ones . . . as time went on, and the unspoken and mysterious 'list' of proscribed vocabulary continued to grow, musicians found themselves with an ever-decreasing pool of words for self-expression at their disposal."

One day the singer's sister's ex-boyfriend, the son of someone in the regime, saw Piero's name on a list. Knowing he was about to be arrested, Piero fled to Panama—that country's leftist military leader, Omar Torrijos, was a close friend who knew Piero's songs by heart. From there, he made his way to Italy before finally settling in Spain, in a small town near Madrid. He made little new music, instead spending his time farming and meditating. After the junta instituted limited reforms, he returned home to Argentina in 1981, his militancy softened by a commitment to nonviolence and a growing interest in Eastern religion. Some of his former fans were disgusted that the onetime troubadour of revolution was now singing songs such as "Manso y tranquilo" ("Meek and Quiet"). Still, he reestablished himself, forming a new band called Prema, a Sanskrit word that means "love," and finding legions of new, younger fans.

Prema's guitar player was fascinated by Sai Baba, and in 1983 he invited Piero to a seminar being given by a devotee from India, a female yoga master. "And that," said Piero, "is where I fell in love with Mataji."

It was Indra Devi's second visit to Argentina. She'd first come for three weeks in 1982, accepting an invitation from a local Sai Baba center. At the time, the country was in the middle of the calamitous Falklands War with Britain, which would soon lead to the fall of Argentina's dictatorship. She'd adored Buenos Aires, finding it at once melancholy and exuberant, an outpost of old Europe on the tip of South America. The city adored her back. Argentineans have always been uniquely introspective—the country has far more psychotherapists and psychoanalysts per capita than any other, the United States included. The blood-drenched insanity of the dictatorship—particularly in a country that had prided itself on its First World sophistication—had left people traumatized and reeling, desperate for spiritual solace. Piero was far from alone in his recent embrace of Eastern mysticism.

When Devi spoke, more than eight hundred people showed up to hear her, those who couldn't fit in the auditorium milling around outside. Afterward, people rushed forward to hug her and kiss her face. It was as if she were being passed from one set of arms to another, floating in a sea of affection and gratitude. In all her eighty-three years, she had never experienced anything comparable.

Thus when Baba's Argentinean devotees invited her to return the next year, just before she left the organization, she happily agreed. She stayed with a wealthy couple, Hugo and Elsa Baldi, and their daughter Francesca, all Sai Baba devotees. After her talk in Buenos Aires, she was to join them in the picturesque lakeside city of Bariloche, at the foot of the Andes. They invited Piero to come along.

She and the singer, then in his thirties, with a handsome face half hidden behind oversize glasses and a long mop of curly brown hair, quickly bonded on the short flight. He plied her with questions about yoga and Hindu philosophy, especially reincarnation. Did she believe in it?

"Of course," she said. How else to explain the world's injustices, why some die in infancy and others live to eighty, why some deserving people are destitute and cruel people wealthy? She had never entertained the idea of a universe without a guiding morality, and to her, only reincarnation provided a satisfactory way to understand the persistence of suffering and evil.

Piero was eager to accept this. Two years earlier, his youngest son, Mariano, had died in infancy, and Piero cherished thoughts about the child's return. Talking to Devi left him elated. She seemed angelic. He asked if she wanted to hear him sing, and she agreed. They flew together from Bariloche to a concert he had scheduled in the city of Tucumán.

She'd known Piero was a musician, but she hadn't realized that he was a star, and the size of the crowd, at least ten thousand people, stunned her. So did the connection between Piero and his audience, their electric fervor. "[Y]ou have a responsibility," she told him afterward. "You have to give them something for their energy. Something positive."

From Tucumán, they went to Salta, where fifteen thousand people showed up for an outdoor concert. After performing "Miedo niño," a song of encouragement to a scared child, Piero asked his new friend to join him onstage so he could introduce her to his fans. Taking the microphone, Devi told the audience, "You have to do what Piero says and fly! You have to detach and fly!" Then, as he sang, the tiny old woman in the sari leapt from the stage and into the upraised arms below. People screamed in delight, passing her over their heads. At the next two concerts, she did the same thing. Piero was amazed. "She loved it!" he said. "She loved it!"

When Devi left, Piero took her admonition seriously. He didn't want to return to political activism, but he wanted to do something to help heal the world. Thus was born Fundación Buenas Ondas, or "Good Vibrations Foundation," a network of loosely organized groups that would simply perform acts of service. Rather than fighting for any sort of ideology, people would come together to sweep the streets, build schools in poor neighborhoods, and visit hospitals and prisons. The groups also meditated together, and Piero wanted Devi to teach them yoga. In August he wrote her a letter telling her that Argentina needed her. She wrote him back, telling him to meet her in Los Angeles the next month for a trip to Egypt.

Devi had always wanted to go there; it was one of her last unfulfilled ambitions. She'd been inspired to take the journey by Paul Brunton's book *A Search in Secret Egypt*, in which he writes of a nighttime vigil in the Great Pyramid of Giza, where he struggles against malevolent forces before coming face-to-face with the luminous spirits of ancient Egyptian priests bearing secrets from the lost city of Atlantis. To help her get there, Bettina Biggart, who was working as a travel agent, had put together a yoga cruise down the Nile, where Devi could teach and travel for free.

Devi was bringing a small entourage with her, mostly women who'd studied with her in Tecate or accompanied her to India to meet Sai Baba. (Her husband would remain with hired aides in Sri Lanka.) Among the travelers was Shama, formerly Maggi Calhoun, a ravishing raven-haired woman who had abandoned a career as an aspiring actress after discovering her psychic abilities. A Baba devotee, Shama had heard about Devi's school in India in the late 1970s and volunteered to collect clothes for the children. She and Devi started writing letters to each other—Shama was deeply moved by Devi's salutation, "Dear Unknown Friend"—then met in person when Devi came to speak at one of the Sai Baba centers in Los Angeles.

"The first time I met her I was so enamored with her," said Shama. "She said, 'Will you drive me to Ojai tomorrow?' I said, 'I'd drive you to the moon!'"

Devi, who had always loved talking to mediums, was tremendously impressed with Shama's abilities. Shama never claimed to be able to read minds or see the future at will; rather, she said, her visions came in sudden flashes. She was, if nothing else, persuasive. In the 1970s, she'd dazzled researchers at the UCLA Parapsychology Laboratory, run by an eccentric psychology professor out of the school's Neuropsychiatric Institute. There, she says, she consulted on murder and missing persons cases for the FBI and the Los Angeles Police Department. Devi raved about her to everyone she knew. She couldn't wait to introduce her to Piero.

Shama saw a strange, inexplicable sort of love affair blooming between the old lady and the crooner. "He was like her pet project, the son she never had, the love she never had in her youth," Shama said. Shama did a reading and determined that Piero had been Devi's father in a past life—and in Egypt, no less! Now Devi and Piero were returning there together. In their deep, mystical friendship, the universe assumed a pleasing, reassuring symmetry.

The trip was a joy, with yoga classes in the morning and a packed itinerary of sightseeing in the afternoon. Inside the Great Pyramid of Giza, Piero played guitar and recorded Devi talking about her life. They hoped to spend the night there just as Brunton had, but couldn't get the necessary permission. They left vowing to return.

After that, Devi started spending more and more of her time with Piero in Argentina; however, with her ailing husband still holding on in Sri Lanka, she couldn't officially move. Though she rarely stayed with Dr. Knauer for long, the idea of his dying alone haunted her. She'd never admit to feeling anything as dull and unproductive as guilt, but she badgered Shama with questions: "Will I be there when he dies? Will I? Will I? I have to be there!" Shama couldn't answer. Yet despite her concern, Devi seemed to live on planes, gleefully telling Shama about practicing headstands in the aisle.

In the end, when Dr. Knauer finally slipped away on the night of December 20, 1984, Devi was at home with him, though not at his side. By then, he was in so much pain that he'd accepted morphine injections, and during his last few days, he hardly spoke. He died quietly; Devi realized he was gone only when one of the nurses she'd hired went into his room and found him completely still.

Anthroposophists believe that it takes three days after death for the etheric body, the life force that animates the physical body, to dissolve fully. During that time, the disembodied self reviews his or her entire life. So Devi, in keeping with her husband's beliefs, some of which, over their marriage, she'd come to share, left his corpse untouched for three days. She surrounded his bed with candles; played Mozart, Bach, and Beethoven (his favorite composers); and kneeled by his side, whispering words of comfort to ease his journey away from this world.

Shama had once asked Dr. Knauer what his life was like with the legendary Indra Devi. "My life with Indra Devi?" he replied, a hint of joking incredulity in his voice. "Most of the time she was gone!" Their separations had pained him far more than her. Now that he was gone, though, she felt the loss acutely.

After three days, she emerged to plan her husband's cremation. The funeral was held in Sri Lanka. Unable to bear the sight of his casket, Devi pasted pieces of paper to the inside of a pair of sunglasses and then wore these blackout shades as she stood at the back of the church. "It was the only time she ever, ever, ever said anything vulnerable in all the years I knew her," said Shama. "When he died she said to me, 'Shama, I feel so alone.'"

Yet being alone also meant being free. "I had the possibility of determining a new course for my life," she wrote. She was eighty-five and ready to start over one last time. On February 15, 1985, she flew to Buenos Aires to settle in Argentina for good.

She moved in with Francesca Baldi, who took charge of organizing her activities. It wasn't easy work—part diva and part incorrigibly free spirit, Devi wouldn't let herself be bound by anything as banal as schedules or appointments. Once, Francesca arranged for her to give a talk in the province of Santa Fe, but at the last minute, Devi decided she'd rather spend a few days at Piero's farm in Cardales, a village outside Buenos Aires. Francesca had to scramble to find a replacement. Devi was sympathetic but unapologetic. She always, Baldi wrote, followed her instinct for "adventure and independence."

Piero's farm, covered with eucalyptus trees, was often her refuge. He'd bought it as part of his Fundación Buenas Ondas, turning it into a bucolic retreat for street kids and those who'd been in trouble with the law. It included classrooms and workshops where the children would study agriculture and ecology. On Saturdays, Devi gave yoga classes, sometimes staying over in a small room that Piero kept just for her. She loved lying beneath the trees, watching their branches sway in the wind and the clouds drift by overhead. Sometimes she would throw her arms around a eucalyptus trunk, the thin skin of her cheek pressed against the bark, trying to hear the tree's vibrations. Often she rolled in the grass like a little girl.

In Buenos Aires, she initially taught in borrowed studios, until she and Francesca Baldi bought a place on Calle Azcuénaga in the stylish Recoleta neighborhood. A journalist visited one of Devi's classes the day after her eighty-sixth birthday and noted that she showed no signs of enervation: "She is restless; constantly moving with coordinated, targeted and expressive gestures; she expresses each word with her body, completely in control of it."

Devi's partnership with Francesca didn't last. The younger woman was still a Sai Baba devotee, and though Devi continued, in some ways, to venerate her former guru—she never stopped believing that he had supernatural powers—his organization regarded her as an apostate. According to Devi, Francesca was forced to choose between them and so severed their partnership just a few months after it began. Devi was, as ever, unruffled. She knew someone else would come along to take care of things. The world had always conspired to spare her from paying attention to life's quotidian details. Why would it stop now?

Sure enough, a young couple named David and Iana Lifar soon stepped in. Devi had first met them when Iana attended one of her talks in Buenos Aires. At the time, the young woman was mired in a crushing depression following a series of health problems—the lecture was the first thing in ages she'd shown any interest in. When it was over and Devi was making her way through a crowd of admirers, a little boy with developmental difficulties, left by his mother to play nearby, took off one of his shoes and sent it flying through the air. It hit Iana on the head in a place where she'd recently had stitches, and she burst into tears.

Devi took Iana in her arms, murmuring "niña querida" ("dear girl"). Iana's family was from Russia, and she thanked Devi in her mother tongue. The sound of the language awakened Devi's affections—this skinny, lost, blue-eyed young woman with pale skin and pretty, soft Slavic features reminded Devi of her long-ago self. Devi instructed her to start practicing yoga and promised to make her a disciple. Iana was overcome, but at first lassitude got the better of her, and she ignored Devi's advice. Two weeks later, she received a letter from Devi checking on her progress. Ashamed that she hadn't made any, she went to the Sai Baba center, where a hatha yoga course was being offered. Soon she was a self-described fanatic.

Initially David Lifar, who was running an import-export business, saw Devi as a sweet old lady, nothing more. The son of a Jewish immigrant from Poland, he was far more interested in politics than religion. Gradually, however, she worked her impish magic on him. In 1987 she had planned to meet Iana in Punta del Este, a resort city on the coast of Uruguay, where she was scheduled to give several presentations. At the last minute, the person who was supposed to handle the logistics couldn't go, and David, organized and practical, stepped in.

All the events went smoothly, and when she was done, Devi asked

David to set up one more: a visit to a prison. In the last decades of her life, Devi made a point of visiting prisoners whenever she could. After all, who was in greater need of techniques for relaxation and mastering the mind? David, curious to see a prison from the inside, agreed to help.

By the time they arrived, the guards had gathered a group of inmates to meet them, telling the prisoners that a "very important person" was coming. The prisoners looked at the beaming old woman with contemptuous hostility. When she started talking, there was derisive laughter.

Then, saying that she was going to show them the power of words, she performed a demonstration, one she often did before a skeptical audience. After coaxing a reluctant volunteer from among her surly listeners, she asked him to hold his arms straight out and keep them there while she attempted to force one of them down. Before trying, she heaped praise on her subject, telling him that he was good, generous, beloved, and able to accomplish what he wanted in life. When she pulled on his right arm with all her might, he resisted easily.

Then she repeated the exercise, but this time, she insulted and mocked the man. She called him a selfish drunk who had mistreated his wife, his children, and even animals. She told him that nobody loved him and that he would always be unhappy. Then she pulled on his right arm again, and it fell easily.

Our thoughts, she told the prisoners, shape our reality. They can make us strong or weak.

The men were astonished and had her try again with a particularly burly, intimidating inmate. Utterly self-assured, Devi pelted the menacing man with calumnies, and then forced his giant arm down. Now the inmates were paying attention, and thirty or forty followed her outside for a yoga class and a short meditation. Their eyes closed, they repeated after her: "I am light. I am love. I have in my heart the divine spark that is God." As they breathed deeply and slowly, the edgy, caged aggression among them evanesced, replaced, for a moment, by tranquility. Devi circulated among them, caressing their heads. When the practice was finished, she hugged and kissed each of the men. Some of them started to cry. At that moment, David Lifar realized he wanted to help her however he could.

Soon David was handling all the practical matters of Devi's life, which was as hectic as ever. She continued to travel incessantly—with the world on the cusp of an unprecedented yoga boom, she was widely in demand. The year after the prison visit, she and David would inaugurate the Fundación Indra Devi, a yoga school. Eventually, it would grow to encompass six studios throughout Buenos Aires. There was just one more big adventure first.

N OCTOBER 1986, Piero took Devi to meet an old friend, Panamanian colonel Roberto Díaz Herrera, at a suite at the Buenos Aires Sheraton. The colonel and his wife, Maigualida, had taken a Boeing 727 from Panama's air force and flown to Argentina on vacation, hoping to escape, at least for a little while, the political intrigue and suffocating anxiety at home. In Panama, Díaz Herrera was, at least nominally, the second-in-command to strongman Manuel Noriega, but he knew that Noriega didn't trust him and that he was on the way out. Already high-strung, Díaz Herrera had felt his nerves flayed. He took tranquilizers, and sometimes he locked himself in his office and wept. Arriving in Buenos Aires, he and his wife had gone on a bit of a bender, and the sitting room Devi entered was strewn with empty champagne bottles and drained whiskey glasses.

Devi, who always enjoyed the company of powerful men, took to the colonel right away. At five foot four (an inch shorter than Noriega), Díaz Herrera was known behind his back as *el enano*, "the midget." He had a handsome face, though, and unlike his shy, introverted boss, he was charming and loquacious, a born storyteller with a gift for mimicry. There was, Devi told him later, "something I really liked about you. There is no logical explanation. It was just a feeling."

Initially, however, the feeling wasn't mutual. In no mood to entertain a white-haired *anciana*, Díaz Herrera went into the bedroom to get Maigualida. "Help me take care of this old lady," he pleaded. Tired, she refused. So Díaz Herrera walked back out, poured himself a highball, and made conversation. Very quickly, he found himself captivated.

The colonel had always scorned the occult superstitions that pervaded Panamanian politics. His boss, Noriega, practiced Santería, believed in astrology, and consulted a longhaired Brazilian psychic named Ivan Trilha, but Díaz Herrera had no time for such peasant notions. Yet Devi, he quickly realized, was no low-rent village sorceress—she was an aristocrat, a woman who'd known Jawaharlal Nehru and Anastas Mikoyan, as well as all sorts of Hollywood legends. She was at once radiantly calm and playful—he would later describe her as "an enlightened piece of the universe that got into the body of a wonderful goblin." He had been desperate to relax. Here, it seemed, was someone who could help him.

They talked for hours. Near midnight, as Devi tried to explain *prana*, she asked if there was any fruit around. There were a few leftover slices of apple on a room service tray, which she said would be good enough. She instructed Díaz Herrera to stand with his arms outstretched and she placed an apple slice in his left hand. Then, in a demonstration like the one she'd performed in the Uruguayan prison, she told him to clench his fists while she tried as hard as she could to push down his right arm. Devi was strong for an eighty-seven-year-old woman, but Díaz Herrera was able to resist.

Next, she replaced the apple slice with a piece of white bread—a dead, impure substance, she said. Once again, she told Díaz Herrera to try to keep his arm raised while she attempted to force it down. It collapsed; he couldn't do it. Astonished, he burst out laughing. They repeated the exercise with a cigarette. Again, his arm fell. This, she said, was *prana*. Pure things give off positive energy; impure things don't. For Díaz Herrera, the effect was world-shaking.

"At that moment there was a connection," he said. "It was the beginning of a love story with a spiritual component." It wasn't just that Devi had charmed him. Noriega had his dark magic—perhaps *prana* could give Díaz Herrera the strength he needed to overcome his adversary. It was the start of what the colonel would later call La Guerra Esotérica, or "The Esoteric War."

Díaz Herrera had already tried to get rid of Noriega by more prosaic means. In 1985, when Noriega was out of the country, he attempted a coup, ordering troops into the capital and trying to turn key colonels against their leader. Yet the CIA, which kept Noriega on the payroll and used him to funnel money and weapons to the Contras in Nicaragua, tipped him off that there was a plot afoot. It almost certainly would have failed anyway—the other colonels depended on Noriega's largesse. "Díaz Herrera had a silvery tongue, but Noriega had a Midas touch," writes journalist Frederick Kempe. When it became clear that Noriega wasn't going anywhere, the shrewd Díaz Herrera managed to deflect blame for the attempted betrayal onto the country's figurehead president, Nicolás Ardito Barletta.

Barletta, who owed his position to an election that Díaz Herrera and Noriega fixed, was forced out. Díaz Herrera stayed put. At first, Noriega saw him as a sort of insurance policy. The colonel was a cousin of former Panamanian leader Omar Torrijos, a widely adored populist who died in a 1981 plane crash. Like Torrijos, he was a left-wing social democrat. As long as Díaz Herrera was Noriega's number two, the Americans couldn't turn on their client without risking handing power to a purported socialist. Yet Díaz Herrera knew that Noriega suspected him, and the atmosphere at the Comandancia, the headquarters of the Panamanian Defense Force, was tense and menacing.

Slowly, Noriega started freezing Díaz Herrera out. He confined him to a desk job, excluded him from important meetings, and dismissed any advice he offered. He warned the colonel's mistresses away and refused to let him travel to barracks outside the capital, where he could solidify his relationships with local commanders. He spread rumors that the Americans believed that Díaz Herrera had murdered opposition leader Hugo Spadafora, a dashing physician and guerrilla fighter, the previous year.

Just before he was killed, Spadafora had returned to Panama from exile in Costa Rica, threatening to reveal Noriega's epic corruption, particularly his involvement in drug and arms trafficking. When Spadafora's body was found—he'd been tortured, mutilated, and beheaded—it created a national and international uproar. Did Noriega intend to pin the crime on the colonel?

Díaz Herrera felt backed into a corner, unsure of his options. After meeting Devi, he grasped at her teachings like a mystical lifeline.

At the time, Shama happened to be in Buenos Aires. She was the latest of Devi's protégés to try to write Devi's biography and had gone to conduct interviews. Soon, though, like Paul O'Brien, she gave up on getting her friend to sit still long enough to unspool her story in a clear, linear way. Besides, her own schedule quickly filled up—Devi had told many people about Shama's abilities, and she found herself agreeing to give reading after reading, using an interpreter for those who didn't speak English. After seeing six people a day for six days straight, Shama was utterly drained. So when Díaz Herrera tried to make an appointment, she told him she was taking that day, a Sunday, off.

He told Shama that he was leaving the next day and absolutely had to have a reading. She replied that she was sorry, but she was exhausted and was heading to a girlfriend's house for lunch. "I didn't realize you don't say no to a Latin leader," she said.

Somehow, he figured out where she was and showed up at her friend's apartment. "My girlfriend opens the door, and in walks Díaz Herrera with all his secret service men, with an open bottle of vodka," Shama recalled. He seemed roguishly charming rather than menacing. "He had this personality that was so charismatic, you couldn't say no," said Shama. "He had that smile like Desi Arnaz. He was very short, not threatening—if anything, just the opposite."

He, meanwhile, was instantly taken with the intense, dark-haired beauty—with her pale skin and straight, heavy bangs, she looked, he said, like Liz Taylor in *Cleopatra*. Later, he told friends she was the most exotic woman he had ever met. He called her "La Gringa."

She agreed to give him a reading, with her hostess acting as an interpreter. First, she had him stare at a spot between and slightly above her beautiful eyes, where the mystical third eye is believed to reside. For nearly two minutes they sat silently while she investigated his aura.

Then, suddenly, she seemed alarmed. "Oh my God, who are you?" she asked him. The vision that came upon her was one of the strongest she'd ever had. "You have a big mission in life," she told him. "A big cause is calling upon you for your help. It involves tens of thousands of people, maybe millions. There's a big plot right now to diminish you." He would be involved in a huge fight, she continued. "Don't expect to win in the short run. You should be prepared to be seen by the world as having lost the fight. You'll think you're going to die, but you will not die."

Fortified by the vodka, Díaz Herrera wasn't that frightened. "I just kept staring at this beautiful gringa," he said. "I just wanted to invite her to bed." But the idea that it was his destiny to confront Noriega took root in his churning mind.

On the way home, Díaz Herrera studied a book that Devi had given him, a Spanish translation of Samuel Sandweiss's *The Holy Man . . . and the Psychiatrist*. Devi may have moved away from the Sai Baba organization, but she still believed in Baba's abilities—indeed, she'd told the Panamanian colonel and his wife all about Baba's many miracles. Sandweiss's book made a powerful impression on Díaz Herrera. *"What good is it to dabble among the waves near the shore, and swear that the sea has no pearls in it and that all tales about them are false?"* Sandweiss quotes Sai Baba (italics in original). To realize Baba's gifts, a devotee had to dive deep. Díaz Herrera was about to take the plunge.

Returning to Panama, Díaz Herrera seemed to lose interest in everything but his own spiritual development. Believing that he could meditate more easily if he were lighter, he went on a diet and grew gaunt. Sometimes he'd sit silently at his desk, his faraway eyes seeming lost in thought. When other officers stared at him, he'd snap, "A little session of meditation wouldn't hurt you." He kept bananas in his office to perform Devi's *prana* demonstration for anyone who was interested, and for some who weren't.

Díaz Herrera set up a Sai Baba temple in his home, and in February 1987 he sent for Shama, enlisting his English-speaking friend José de Jesús "Chuchú" Martínez to make the arrangements. An orthodox Marxist and Sorbonne-trained mathematician, Chuchú thought Díaz Herrera had lost his mind. If this was what things had come to—American psychics!—the whole country was doomed. Still, Chuchú was loyal, and ultimately he did as he was asked.

At first, Shama said no. When Díaz Herrera, speaking through Chuchú, insisted, she said she'd consult her master, Sai Baba. The next day, she told them that she'd received a message from the avatar, and that they could send her a ticket to Panama City. It was the first of several trips over the course of the year. Most of the time she came alone, though once, at Díaz Herrera's request, she brought a nutritionist specializing in a New Age therapy called psychokinesiology.

"He put me up in an incredible penthouse apartment," said Shama. "Every time I went there I was just treated like Princess Diana. They were so nice to me it was incredible." As soon as she arrived the first time, she went to Díaz Herrera's powder-blue mansion in the ritzy suburban neighborhood of Altos del Golf ("Golf Heights"), not far from where Noriega lived. Protected by high white walls, the mansion was adorned by four Grecian columns and two sphinxes. There was a grand two-story entryway, marble floors throughout, and a swimming pool in the big emerald yard shaded by lush vegetation. Inside, Shama said, she would give everybody readings, "the whole family, even second cousins. It was all such an incredible joyous adventure."

For Panamanians, it was quite a bit more than that. Shama told Díaz Herrera that in a past life he had been the nineteenth-century

Russian writer Alexander Pushkin. Looking him up in the encyclopedia, Díaz Herrera discovered that his former self had been a great romantic idealist. About more urgent matters, Shama, after seeing a photo of Noriega, told her host, "Noriega is your enemy. He is the man I was talking about in Buenos Aires. He is evil, and he will do anything in his power to destroy you."

To Díaz Herrera, her abilities were indisputable. How else could this woman from California so fully comprehend Noriega? Every time they spoke, he would try to extract more and more details of what he was up against. She was, he said, "like military intelligence, psychic military intelligence."

Maybe he had disdained such things before, but no more. After all, he'd read that the Soviets were doing tests to find proof of telepathy, and they were atheists! If the world's most committed materialists took psychic powers seriously as a tool in the Cold War, surely such powers could help him.

He would need to relax and focus. To help with that, he invited Devi to Panama City. She was delighted to come—it would give her the opportunity to spread the message of yoga to yet another country. The colonel installed her in his mother-in-law's house, next door to his own. His office took charge of her daily schedule, setting up TV interviews and visits to charities and a children's hospital. He arranged for her to deliver a speech at a local university and introduced her to the packed audience.

She tried to teach Díaz Herrera how to breathe, putting his hands on her belly so he could feel the expansion when she inhaled deeply. But he was a very busy man, and as much as he admired her, he found it hard, at first, to give her his undivided attention.

One day, she rang his buzzer just as he was heading out. She gave him a long, tight, silent hug. He hugged her back but was impatient; his car was waiting for him. "You're leaving?" she said sweetly. "When are you going to be able to give me three minutes, without a telephone, without anybody calling you?"

He smiled—she wasn't an easy person to say no to. "Fifteen minutes," he said.

"Oooh," she replied, her face alight, "fifteen minutes! We can do marvels in fifteen minutes!"

They went into his room. She took his hand, transmitting, he said, maternal love. Then she gave him what felt like an initiation.

Many years before, Sai Baba had given her a gaudy ring with a sapphire surrounded by seven diamond-tipped golden rays. Having long ago given up jewelry, she didn't particularly like the ring, though she didn't say anything to Baba. The next day, he asked for it back, put it in his palm, and blew. When he opened his hand, there was a diamond solitaire in its place. "Every time you wish, you will see me in the ring, but no one else will," he said.

Throughout everything that had happened—her infatuation with Premananda, her break with the Sai organization, her move to Argentina—Devi had never taken the ring off. Now she used it to bless the man who hoped to bring down Noriega. Through the ring, she said, Sai Baba was offering the colonel a mantra. She put her hands on Díaz Herrera's head while she said it: "Rama, Rama, Rama." (As an avatar of Vishnu, Rama exemplified courage and honor.) Díaz Herrera closed his eyes and repeated: "Rama, Rama, Rama."

He started talking to her about his battle with Noriega—how outraged he was by the dictator's rampant criminality, how desperate he was to overthrow him, how helpless he felt in the wake of his failed coup attempt. It was like a confession. "What do I do with this man?" he asked. "What do I do with him?"

"The only thing I can tell you to do is to visualize him, shut your eyes, and send him love and light," she said.

"How can I send him light and love?" asked Díaz Herrera, indignant.

"But then," she continued, "take the decision to act according to your conscience."

It was as if she were sanctifying his dream of revolution. Her words, he said, were a two-sided message: "Love and light, but throw him out."

They spoke more: of life and death, karma and dharma. When

they emerged after an hour and a half, he was completely relaxed. "I left there on a different frequency," he said. "We had a tremendous love. Besides my mother, nobody has loved me like Mataji. Nobody."

A few days later, Devi asked Díaz Herrera if she could accompany him to his office. He tried to put her off—he adored her, but he was also a little bit embarrassed to be seen with her in front of his military colleagues.

"You're going to be bored," he told her.

"No, no[,] I want to go," she replied. "I'm not going to bother you. [T]ake me to your office."

All the way there, she held his hand in the backseat. He felt the eyes of his bodyguards watching them in the rearview mirror, and he knew they thought he'd gone mad.

At the office, she sat on a couch while he attended to some paperwork. It didn't take her long, he said, to win over all his secretaries and every military man who passed through. "She was very magnetic and attractive, and the people who would see her smile, even though they didn't know who she was, felt that they were in front of a great person, an exquisite woman," he said.

Noriega, of course, heard all about it. Word came to Díaz Herrera that the dictator had been asking, "Who does Roberto have in his office, a psychic and a yogi?" For the colonel, this was not necessarily a bad thing. The dictator believed in this stuff. Perhaps he would be intimidated by the spiritual firepower his rival was amassing.

Díaz Herrera continued to squire his spiritual adviser around town. He took her as his date to a dinner party on an Italian cruise ship, where she performed a mind-over-matter demonstration on the ship's burly Russian captain. Enlisting three other petite ladies, they each put two fingers underneath him and, imagining him to be as light as a feather, lifted him up. This is, of course, a classic girls' slumber party game, but neither Díaz Herrera nor the captain was ever a little girl, and they were flabbergasted. Devi was the star of the evening.

Most nights, Devi dined at Díaz Herrera's home, and after dinner she'd lead the couple and a few close friends in meditation. During these sessions, she'd expound on the dangers of materialism and the necessity of detachment. She repeated a parable that Sai Baba often told. "When a peasant wants to catch a monkey, he uses a big pot with a narrow mouth as a trap," the swami once said. "Inside the pot, he puts edibles which the monkey loves. The monkey finds the pot and puts its paws inside it to grasp as much of the stuff as he can hold. Once it does so, it is unable to pull out its paws from the small mouth of the pot. The monkey imagines that someone inside the pot is holdings its paws, so it struggles and attempts to run away with the pot, only to fail and get trapped. No one is holding the monkey; it has trapped itself because of its greed."

So, too, were people bound by their fear of losing their material possessions. "The moment you give up the pleasures and detach yourself, you will be free," said Devi. The story had a striking impact on Díaz Herrera. He was hardly innocent of the regime's corruption. His chateau and Mercedes had been bought with the money he'd made selling Panamanian visas to Cuban émigrés. He had relished the perquisites of power, but if he was truly going to take on Noriega, he had to make his peace with losing them. He still hoped he wouldn't have to, but he was getting ready.

Then Devi returned to Buenos Aires having set in motion events that would change Latin American history.

Contrary to Díaz Herrera's hopes, word of his new metaphysical reinforcements failed to cow the dictator. Certainly Noriega had been momentarily unnerved, but Trilha, his psychic, assured him that he had nothing to fear. "Trilha showed Noriega on an astrological map that, as an Aquarius, he had a strong field of protection and mental clarity that Díaz Herrera lacked," wrote Kempe. So rather than placating his second-in-command, Noriega spurned him even more. He'd briefly considered a plan to rid himself of Díaz Herrera by making him ambassador to Japan, a prestigious and lucrative position. Instead, deciding it was no longer worth the trouble of keeping him around, he simply retired him.

For three days after he was cashiered, Díaz Herrera tried frantically to reach his old boss, but Noriega dodged him. Finally, Díaz Herrera had his guard deliver a handwritten note to Noriega's house. "You want to begin a total war with me, and I am trying to avoid it, for Lorena, Sandra, and Thais," wrote the colonel, referring to Noriega's daughters. "But I am not afraid of you. If you don't talk to me, you are going to confront a total war on my behalf. Don't run away from me. Call me." He heard nothing.

"Now," said Díaz Herrera, "my plan was to make Panama explode. I had to shake everybody like an earthquake." He'd tried to defeat Noriega militarily and failed. He would need to win over the minds of the people. He could denounce Noriega, but he knew that he was himself regarded as no better than an accomplice. He would have to make a grand gesture, to show a willingness to make real sacrifices, to renounce his monkey-like attachment to the spoils of corruption.

On June 6, Díaz Herrera told the editor of the anti-Noriega newspaper *La Prensa* that if he sent a journalist to the colonel's house, he would make some stunning disclosures. The editor was skeptical, but a reporter and photographer were dispatched anyway. When they arrived, they found the colonel under a sort of spell. First, he made a confession. He'd helped rig the 1984 election, he said—the final details of the plan had been arranged right there, in his own home. That home, further, was half-stolen, bought largely with Cuban bribes. Finally, he admitted, he'd helped force President Barletta out, twisting his arm—he mimicked the gesture—when he resisted.

Then came a fusillade of accusations. Noriega, he said, was responsible for Spadafora's murder. The dictator had stolen the twelve million dollars that the Shah of Iran had paid to Torrijos in exchange for giving him refuge after Iran's revolution. Most shockingly of all, Díaz Herrera accused Noriega of working with the CIA to kill Torrijos by putting a bomb on his plane.

What Díaz Herrera was doing was unprecedented. "The Godfather's second-in-command was ratting on the mafia," wrote Kempe.

Journalists, supporters, and curious onlookers flocked to his house, where the colonel repeated his charges to anyone who cared to listen. Among them was Winston Spadafora, brother of Hugo, who had dedicated himself to finding justice for his murdered sibling. Díaz Herrera started referring to his home as the "headquarters of dignity." He stood outside, giving out photocopies of handwritten anti-Noriega pronouncements that recipients were supposed to duplicate and pass on. One of these screeds referred to Noriega as Cain, sinful brother of the biblical Abel.

The middle-class people massing in the suburban streets of Altos del Golf were not accustomed to blatant shows of political violence. Panama was a placid country; when Noriega used force, he did so behind the scenes. Thus the people outside Díaz Herrera's mansion were shocked when black-clad riot police in storm trooper helmets appeared on the scene and attacked the crowd with bird shot and teargas. It was, wrote Kempe, their "political baptism."

Protests spread all over the country in response to Díaz Herrera's charges—though, for a would-be revolution, it was a bizarrely tame and bourgeois one, led by middle-class Rotary Club types who were no longer able to tolerate rule by an uncouth and epically corrupt thug. Demonstrations often happened during lunchtime and cocktail hour. "It's like watching your mom and dad riot at the mall," wrote *Rolling Stone*'s P. J. O'Rourke.

This does not, however, mean that the standoff wasn't serious. Amid intensifying violence, Noriega declared a state of emergency and suspended the constitution's civil liberties provisions. Opposition newspapers were shut down. More than fifteen hundred protesters were arrested. Some were tortured, and more were tossed into fetid, filthy cells with the general prison population, who had tacit permission to rough them up. There were rumors that Noriega was arranging to have dissidents raped by carriers of HIV.

The violence put the United States, Noriega's patron, in a difficult spot. "In the good old days in Panama, nobody seemed to mind that the military ran the nation; that elections were routinely rigged to place the Panamanian Defense Force's candidate in the presidential palace; that banks laundered millions of dollars of Colombian cocaine money; that business people with the right connections made fortunes selling U.S. goods to Cuba, circumventing the U.S. trade embargo," wrote the *Miami Herald*'s Andrés Oppenheimer. "Washington dealt with this by looking the other way, content with keeping the strategic Panama Canal immune to the political troubles of neighboring countries. And then Díaz Herrera held his little press conference."

Inside Díaz Herrera's blue chateau, hundreds of people camped out amid the deepening political crisis. Among them were anti-Noriega activists who, only days before, had considered the colonel their enemy. Priests came to serve as human shields; one looked for handcuffs so he could attach himself to Díaz Herrera in the event of a raid. The mood was charged with spiritual fervor. Some supporters rested on prayer rugs unfolded on the lawn. A Panamanian Hindu convert dressed in white robes wandered around chanting mantras.

The colonel, reported the *New York Times*, "sits cross-legged, speaking in cryptic phrases punctuated by long silences. Associates advise visitors that when he feels positive vibrations, his palms face upward; he turns his palms down if questioning becomes too aggressive." Díaz Herrera claimed to be receiving psychic messages directly from Sai Baba. "I have no doubt that he, not I, is in command of everything," he said. At his feet sat a golden plaque with Sai Baba's lotus logo on it.

In the end, they were holed up for six weeks. Just before the military helicopters came on July 27, Díaz Herrera called Shama on a secret line, terrified. "He was like a frightened rabbit calling me: What should I do, what's going to happen?" she said. By then she was scared, too, because Noriega had started sending her letters through the Panamanian consulate instructing her to tell Díaz Herrera to get out of Panama. "I was saying, 'Please, don't drag me into this, because you're putting my life at stake,'" said Shama.

Soon after Díaz Herrera hung up the phone with Shama, elite Israeli-trained troops stormed the mansion, firing Uzis and hurling teargas bombs. They found Díaz Herrera and his wife lying on their bedroom floor. Above them was a photograph of a half-smiling Sai Baba in a saffron robe. The raid lasted less than fifteen minutes. The colonel, his family, and dozens of his supporters were loaded into Panamanian Defense Force vehicles and taken away.

After several days in an undisclosed location, Díaz Herrera issued a statement recanting his accusations against Noriega. (He would later cite an Irish proverb, "It's better to be a coward for one minute, than dead for the rest of your life," attributing it to Napoléon.)

Maigualida and their kids went into exile in Venezuela, where she was from. She lobbied incessantly for her husband's release, enlisting the help of a former Venezuelan president and of politicians in Spain and Peru. After several months, her efforts succeeded, and in December 1987, Díaz Herrera was allowed to join his family in Caracas, where he struggled in his attempts to build a real estate business.

He had failed; Noriega was still in power. Yet far away in Washington, Noriega's support was collapsing. In the wake of the protests, Senator Edward Kennedy submitted a resolution calling for a "public accounting" of the dictator's role in Spadafora's murder and the fixing of the 1984 election, and in drug trafficking and money laundering. The resolution passed 75–13. America's man in Panama had become an embarrassment.

In February 1988, a court in Miami indicted Noriega on twelve counts of narcotrafficking and racketeering. The next year, in Operation Just Cause, American troops invaded Panama. Noriega was deposed, arrested, and brought to the United States for trial. Found guilty, he was imprisoned until 2007 and eventually extradited back to Panama to serve a prison sentence there. By then, Martín Torrijos, Omar's son, was the country's president, and Díaz Herrera was back in government, serving as the Panamanian ambassador to Peru.

"For me, Indra clarified what I knew in my interior consciousness had to be done," Díaz Herrera said in 2013, sitting in the living room of his condo in one of Panama City's new luxury high-rises, a wall of windows looking out over the expanse of the Pacific ocean. Devi gave him, he said, "the courage to confront whatever consequence, because even death is not the end. The spirit goes on."

Shama, it seems, had been right.

HERE IS the last astonishing thing about Indra Devi: she lived, for the most part, happily ever after.

Few biographies have joyous endings, particularly those of pioneering, adventurous women. Even in the best of old ages, there's usually some stoic, bittersweet acceptance of diminishing relevance and attenuated abilities. Yet, fortified by a lifetime of spiritual discipline, Devi largely transcended regret, learning to observe the world's flux with smiling detachment. Further, because she seemed to float through life rather than cling to it, because she was so rarely weak or needy or choked by nostalgia, she never became marginal.

As global interest in yoga exploded in the 1990s, she grew only more famous, her vitality the ultimate testament to the power of the practice. She was adored for many reasons, but among them was the way her very existence suggested that, with the right regimen, one could indeed remain forever young, forever healthy.

Devi enjoyed playing with people's expectations of the old. As an act of service, she visited lonely people in nursing homes—people who were almost all younger than she was. Once, getting off a plane, she was offered a wheelchair. She consented to be pushed in it, but as soon as she reached the arrivals gate, she took off running and giggling.

Another time, she traveled with Piero to Bogotá, Colombia, for a charity concert. After a few songs, he introduced her to the crowd as his master and friend, a woman who'd met Gandhi and Tagore and Krishnamurti. Devi had always refused to safety-pin her sari, insisting on tying it the old-fashioned way, without buttons or clasps. Toward the end of her life she became less dexterous, and her clothing less secure. On this occasion, as she walked onstage, the garment slipped off, leaving her almost naked before thousands of young people, like a scene in a common nightmare. She burst out laughing and, utterly unperturbed, put it back on as she continued talking. She was, marveled Piero, "above everything."

For much of her life, Devi's only goal had been to make yoga known to the West. In the 1990s, as the discipline became a ubiquitous part of cosmopolitan urban culture, signifier of a lifestyle at once wholesome and sexy, her dream was more than fulfilled. In its latest incarnation, yoga is a holistic, authentic alternative to the aerobics boom of the 1980s, more grounded but just as physically challenging and far more fashionable. Throughout the last decade of the twentieth century a parade of celebrities, their star power matching that of Devi's high-wattage Hollywood students, testified to their devotion to the practice—Madonna, Sting, Gwyneth Paltrow, Christy Turlington. In 1998, Madonna released her four-time Grammy-winning *Ray of Light*, a spiritually infused dance record; the track "Shanti/Ashtangi" sets a Sanskrit chant over a deep, jagged bassline. Yoga had arrived at the very center of American popular culture.

The same year that *Ray of Light* came out, New York's chic Jivamukti Yoga Center moved from the still-gritty East Village to a nine-thousand-square-foot emporium above a branch of Crunch gym. "Like some sort of millennial nightclub (there is a waterfall, plastic lotus flowers, a boutique), the fuchsia-and-turquoise Jivamukti studio is perfumed with the promise of pleasure," Penelope Green wrote in the *New York Times*, continuing: "A sense of throbbing expectancy lends a charge to the place, just like at a disco." For a while, it was among the trendiest places in the trendiest city in the world.

Even as yoga assumed a high-fashion gloss, it was also democratized to an unprecedented degree, offered in suburban gyms and, as Devi had once hoped, forward-thinking offices, particularly in Silicon Valley. Four years before Madonna jumped on board, the stodgy *U.S. News & World Report* had already declared "Yoga Goes Mainstream," noting that the number of Americans practicing yoga had doubled in only three years, to an estimated four million.

That number has since quintupled: a 2012 survey commissioned by *Yoga Journal* found that 20.4 million Americans (almost 9 percent of U.S. adults) practiced yoga. Even if a good number of those have only dabbled in it at the gym, it's clear that yoga had become an enormous American phenomenon as well as a global one.

Devi planted the seeds for the yoga boom of the 1990s, training a host of teachers who would soon find themselves with throngs of new students. Yet the yoga that became globally popular in Devi's last years was much more vigorous than the style she taught. Krishnamacharya had trained her in a type of asana practice suited to a middle-aged woman. When she taught sun salutations, she warned practitioners against exhausting themselves and even suggested they take a few minutes of rest immediately afterward. The yoga that spread rapidly in the 1990s, however, was based on a regimen Krishnamacharya developed for young boys, and it was all about testing the body's limits. Sweaty and sometimes punishing, this yoga was, like the old hatha of India's wandering ascetics, a way of mortifying the flesh, though it was often done in the service of beauty rather than ego annihilation.

The man who deserves immediate credit for the new yoga explosion was a student of Krishnamacharya's named Sri K. Pattabhi Jois. The son of a Brahmin astrologer, Jois began studying with Krishnamacharya as a schoolboy. Unlike Iyengar, he thrived under the master's strict discipline and was often called upon to demonstrate advanced postures. In Krishnamacharya's classes for young boys, poses were performed drill-style, linked by *vinyasas*, the flowing series of movements, familiar to most modern yoga students, that takes a practitioner from standing, through the half push-up known as *Chaturanga*, and then into downward-facing dog.

Jois, who grew into a fierce but ebullient master, codified these teachings into a system called ashtanga yoga, in which a series of poses are performed in the same order every day. (There are six progressively more difficult series in the ashtanga system, and very few people have mastered all of them.) This yoga is self-guided—teachers are there to help students learn and perfect the poses, but students move through the routine on their own—and immensely challenging, creating a cultlike intensity among some adepts.

Most people lack the patience and endurance (physical or mental) necessary for a sustained ashtanga practice. In the 1990s, though, many teachers adapted ashtanga methods to create yoga classes offering sweaty workouts, often accompanied by a throbbing pop soundtrack. The power yoga taught in gyms and the flow style popular at fashionable urban studios such as Jivamukti are rooted in Jois's system, even if Jois himself disapproved of would-be innovators. In a 1995 letter to *Yoga Journal*, written in response to a cover story on "Power Yoga," Jois wrote, "I was disappointed to find that so many novice students have taken Ashtanga yoga and have turned it into a circus for their own fame and profit . . . It would be a shame to lose the precious jewel of liberation in the mud of ignorant body building."

No one would confuse Devi's yoga with bodybuilding, which may be why her slower, gentler style fell out of fashion. Teachers whom she trained continue offering classes all over the world, but they're older now, and so, in many cases, are their students.

Yet Indra Devi's spirit animates modern Western yoga, even more so than those of Jois or Iyengar or Bikram Choudhury, the Rolls-Royce-collecting creator of hot yoga. Today in the West, yoga is an overwhelmingly female pursuit—the *Yoga Journal* survey found that 82.2 percent of practitioners are women. It's part of the same cultural matrix as organic food, holistic spas, and biodynamic beauty products—things that seem to go together so naturally that it's easy to forget that they weren't always linked. It was Indra Devi, more than anyone else, who turned a very male discipline into an uplifting ritual for cosmopolitan, spiritual-but-not-religious women.

As a balm for the anxieties inherent in having a changeable and ever-scrutinized female body, yoga has become, among elite women, almost a requisite part of pregnancy, along with designer prenatal yoga clothes that have their direct antecedents in the "lotus suits" created by Devi's students at Page Boy. Devi's instructions for pregnant women in 1963's *Renew Your Life through Yoga*—eat raw foods and juices, exercise daily, practice deep breathing to obviate the need for pain-relieving drugs during labor, make sure to breast-feed—considered quirky at the time, are today conventional wisdom in the circles where yoga is most popular. The lifestyle she promoted—a mash-up of Hindu practices, Western esotericism, health food, show-business glamour, and back-to-nature femininity—has become nearly ubiquitous in privileged circles.

Anyone who practices yoga in the West knows, on some level, that he or she is involved in a hybrid culture. There is an immense gulf between the limber young women in Lululemon yoga gear rolling out rubber mats on the hardwood floors of modern studios and the ash-smeared half-naked yogins who contort themselves on the banks of the Ganges. They exist in two different conceptual universes; though they live in the same time, they're as distant from each other as medieval mendicant monks are from the worshippers in suburban American megachurches. This disconnect makes some people uncomfortable, especially if they turned to yoga precisely because they were looking for something more meaningful and authentic than a gym workout. If yoga isn't just exercise, if it isn't religion, and if it isn't, in its current form, even all that old, then what the hell is it?

Every so often, *Yoga Journal* will run an article expressing worry that the true spirit of yoga is threatened by the practice's exploding popularity. In a 2000 feature asking whether yoga was becoming "too popular for its own good," the scholar Georg Feuerstein was quoted: "Even a tradition like hatha yoga, which had the body as its focus, always had the goal of reaching liberation and enlightenment. This has dropped away from many of the Western schools of yoga." Part of the appeal of ashtanga yoga is the sense that it is real and unadulterated, unlike more fluid, improvisational forms.

Here, however, is a lesson we can take from Devi's life and from the friends, teachers, and gurus who shaped her: There is no such thing as unchanging authenticity. Far from a static repository of ancient wisdom, India is as culturally dynamic as any place on the planet, influencing and being influenced by the West in equal measure. Restless Westerners (and particularly restless Western women) have long gone to India seeking ancient spiritual treasures, only to find themselves instead part of a creative dialogue with people eager to innovate in their own traditions. That dialogue continues today, as practitioners all over the world develop new styles of yoga, which in turn influence the way yoga is practiced on the subcontinent. The *Yoga Journal* story about the Americanization of the practice begins in New Delhi, where the writer's guide, a young woman enamored of self-help, tells her, "I love yoga so much. If only I had enough money, I would go to California to study it."

Some people might find this disillusioning—there's a reason that the relatively recent provenance of so many yoga poses is rarely discussed in yoga studios—but it's also freeing, because it means we don't have to think about yoga in terms of purity and corruption or to feel guilty for adapting it. Indeed, to adapt yoga to modern needs is even to be part of a tradition of sorts. Today's Western yoginis may not really be heiresses to Patanjali, but they are very much part of a lineage that goes back to Madame Blavatsky, Annie Besant, and Indra Devi.

In the last years of her life, Devi came to understand and even appreciate the way that women, following her example, were adopting and transforming techniques developed by Indian male ascetics. "Now that women have liberated themselves from the house, they are looking for something spiritual," she told the *Buenos Aires Herald*. "Men, now that they have lost the prerogatives they had for thousands of years, tend to justify themselves, taking refuge in technology." A few months later, the author of another profile wrote that Devi "perceives a great imbalance between the sexes, and describes men as being on the throne with a choice to make: either step down of their own accord, or be pushed off."

She had become, in the end, a sort of feminist. Though she'd always been apolitical, she started speaking out on one burning issue: abortion rights. Worshipping freedom, she was incensed by the idea that anyone would be forced to bear a baby against her will, and the growing antiabortion movement in the United States left her indignant.

For reasons that were never clear, Devi was also convinced that a douche of coffee and olive oil could bring on a late period. Further, she believed that this secret knowledge could give women control over their bodies. So, in a quixotic attempt to liberate women from the tyranny of biology, she had leaflets typed up in three languages that she would distribute to friends and students. Saying that it was a "gross injustice" that men could force women to continue an unwanted pregnancy, the flyers offered her recipe, and concluded, chain-letter style, by urging recipients to copy them and send them on. That way, eventually, "every woman in the world will be able to get this simple and free information."

Of course, yoga remained her overriding passion, and the worldwide yoga explosion meant that she was in greater demand than ever. In 1988 she joined a host of global yoga luminaries in Zinal, Switzerland, for the inauguration of the International Yoga Federation, a body meant to unite national and regional yoga associations. The same year, she traveled to Madras for Krishnamacharya's onehundredth birthday. There is video of her draping his neck in a garland of flowers and then sitting as his feet as he blesses her. "He likes you," says his smiling son. "I like him too!" she replies, laughing. Together, they chant a Sanskrit mantra, a prayer for mankind to be led from darkness to light, from the fear of death to the knowledge of immortality.

If there was any fear of death left in Devi, she never showed it. A psychic once told her that she would die at ninety, so in 1989 she prepared to say a grand farewell, but the year passed and she was still working as hard as ever, spending her ninety-first birthday in Moscow. There, she was interviewed on a popular television show while sitting, throughout, in lotus pose. The next day, admirers mobbed her on the street. Russia was in the early stages of its own yoga boom—by 2010, the *New York Times* reported, "Yoga, which was officially taboo in Soviet times but retained an underground following, has been embraced by Russia's elite. In 2007, shortly before he became president, [Dmitry] Medvedev told Itogi magazine that he was 'mastering yoga,' as one activity that helps him deal with the stress of political obligations."

Devi was back in India in 1990. There, rushing off a plane in Madras, she fell and broke her arm. A doctor told her that without surgery she would never be able to use it again. Ignoring him, she created a program of rehabilitative exercises for herself and recovered within eight months. The next year, she traveled to India once again, and then, the year after that, to England. In 1995 she joined yoga teachers from all over the world at a conference in Jerusalem designed to bring Jews and Arabs together through the practice.

An old friend of hers, Tao Porchon-Lynch—who, as of this writing, continues to teach surprisingly vigorous classes in her late nineties—remembers hearing her inimitable voice from the back of the stage. "Suddenly, I hear somebody say, 'I can do it! Don't tell me I can't do it!'" says Porchon-Lynch. Someone had made the mistake of trying to help Indra Devi down the stairs.

In 1996 Devi planned to go to India one more time, perhaps for good. Not long after she'd flouted the first prediction of her death by surviving her ninetieth year, she'd gone to see a French psychic living in Buenos Aires, who told her she would die in a year ending in eight. Again, she began preparing for the end. Often she told people that she planned to spend her last years in a hermitage, in keeping with the tradition of many Indian spiritual masters. It would have been her last reinvention: the secluded contemplative.

It's hard to say where she would have gone. Many of her old friends were dead, and her onetime spiritual homes no longer offered refuge. In 1994, Swami Premananda, who had built a new ashram in Tamil Nadu, was arrested for raping and illegally detaining orphan and indigent girls who'd been entrusted to his care and for involvement in the murder of an estranged disciple. Three years later, he was convicted and sentenced to life in prison. (He died behind bars in 2011.) Devi must have been aware of the case, but she never spoke of it publicly.

Meanwhile, whatever faith she'd had left in Sai Baba was destroyed in 1993, when six people were killed in the avatar's residence in circumstances that remain mysterious. A few things are clear: Four young devotees armed with knives had broken into Baba's quarters. When his attendants tried to stop them, the intruders stabbed two of them to death. While Sai Baba escaped through a back stairway, the boys tried to barricade themselves in his bedroom. Then heavily armed police barged in and, citing self-defense, killed the four boys.

After that, things get murky. To this day, no one knows what the boys' motive was, and many have alleged that they were killed to prevent them from testifying, possibly about sexual abuse. Velayudhan Nair, the former home secretary of Andhra Pradesh, claimed there was a cover-up and called the shootings "absolute cold-blooded murder." Some of the policemen involved were arrested, but charges were never brought, and according to a BBC report, Sai Baba was never even interviewed.

In the wake of the killings, Devi told Díaz Herrera, with whom she remained close during his exile, that she was finished with her former guru. "She said there was a crime, but it was covered up," he recalled. "She cut everything off." Despite her aversion to challenging the faith of others, she even broached the subject of the murders with her old friend Bettina Biggart, who was still a Baba devotee and was outraged by Devi's impertinence.

"She was totally in the wrong on that," Biggart said. "She wasn't there, she didn't know what happened. In India, treatment can get a little rough. If she accepts that he was the avatar, you do not question what he does! Whether he's God or the avatar, he's not a normal being, and everything he does is for upliftment!"

For Devi, with so many connections severed, returning to India would have meant, once again, sailing into the unknown. This had never stopped her before, so she boarded a plane, but with a new, unaccustomed unease. There was a layover in Singapore, and while in the airport, she bumped into a door and hurt her finger. The injury, she decided, was a sign that the trip wasn't meant to be. Without leaving the airport, she turned around and went right back to Argentina and the people she loved. She had reached, she realized, her final incarnation, at least in this lifetime.

People sometimes asked her why she never carried out her plan to retire. "I don't know!" she writes. "I didn't want to!" Having never claimed that she was an Eastern spiritual master, she felt no need to abide by traditions of renunciation. "I changed my opinion because there are always more things to do."

Including one more trip. In 1998 Díaz Herrera, by then back in Panama City, got a worried phone call from David Lifar. "Mataji wants to go to Panama to see you," Lifar said. She insisted on traveling alone. She was ninety-nine and had recently had fainting spells, but she would not be dissuaded. So Lifar put her on a 6:00 a.m. flight from Buenos Aires to Lima, Peru, where she had a two-hour layover, finally reaching Panama in the afternoon. Díaz Herrera picked her up at Tocumen airport.

At his house—more modest than the Altos del Golf mansion, which he had long since leased—she took off her sandals. Assuming she was exhausted after the long flight, he asked if she wanted to rest a while.

"If you want to rest, go rest," she said to him.

"No," he said, "If you want to rest a little from the trip . . ."

"If you want to go, my dear, you go," she repeated. "I'm not coming here to rest."

During that trip, he accompanied her on a visit to a hospital for the elderly and once again arranged for her to give a talk at a university. Because 1998 was the year she'd been prophesied to die, Díaz Herrera believed she'd come to say good-bye. She was weaker than she'd been before, the sparkle in her eye not quite as bright, her memory unreliable.

One morning, 9:30 came and she still hadn't gotten out of bed. Worried, Díaz Herrera's wife went to check on her. Walking into Devi's room, she found her sitting up in bed. "Nobody's come to give me my good morning kiss," Devi said sweetly. "How can I get up without my kiss?" Touched, Díaz Herrera went in and gave her a hug. One can see this as senility or playfulness, or both. For the colonel, it was evidence of her capacity for love.

Once again, prophecy failed. The year 1999 arrived, and with it, Devi's one-hundredth birthday. David and Iana Lifar organized a huge party for her in Buenos Aires, and more than three thousand people came to celebrate her century on earth. By that point, her memory had started to go, though only those who'd known her for a long time realized it. Biggart, in town for the festivities, remembered accompanying her to a restaurant. "She was out of it then," she said. "Nobody knew it but Rosita and I." Yet when a group of photographers showed up, Biggart recalled, Devi straightened up and pulled her shoulders back, a grande dame ready for her close-up. She was still present enough to care how she looked in pictures.

Devi had given up teaching, though she continued to give talks to small groups of students. Her eyesight had become bad, but she wouldn't wear glasses, so she didn't do much reading anymore. Often she'd sit in her room listening to music and feeding pigeons from her window.

Her death, when it came in 2002, just before her 103rd birthday, was not a good one. David Lifar told journalists that she "went in peace, without suffering at all," but other friends recall her fury at being confined to a bed in a clinic, fed by a nasogastric tube that she kept trying to pull out. Convinced that she was ready to die, they were outraged at the measures that were taken to sustain her, but lacked the legal standing to do anything about them. "We just have to understand that this is part of Karma, which Mataji had to fulfill in this life," wrote one of her disciples.

In keeping with the teachings Devi had picked up from her husband—as well as her own lifelong fear of being trapped in a coffin before she was fully gone—her corpse was left alone for three days in order for her soul to review the life she'd lived before departing. Perhaps she should have been left for longer, because the story unwinding before her disembodied self—in reverse, according to the Anthroposophists—would have had many more chapters than most.

If the Anthroposophists were right, she would have seen Panama on the cusp of an attempted revolution, Buenos Aires after the dictatorship, and Sri Lanka at the start of the civil war. She'd have watched herself at Sai Baba's ashram during the exhilarating early days when a new epoch in human history seemed to be at hand. She'd have revisited her ranch in Mexico during the height of the counterculture and Hollywood in its lavish heyday. She'd have seen Shanghai during the bleakest days of the war, the Indian independence movement, and the birth of Bollywood. She'd be in Ommen with the Theosophical Society at the moment when it seemed that the Messiah had arrived, and then dancing in the cabarets of Berlin. She'd again flee the terror of the Russian Revolution, and then relive the aborted hope with which it began. Finally, she'd have found herself in the grand brick house by the river in Riga with her adored teenage mother. She would have seen the start of the twenty-first century, the whole of the twentieth, and the end of the nineteenth.

Then, when her self had truly dissolved, her body was cremated and her ashes scattered in the Río de la Plata, trailed by floating South American flowers, their stems trimmed to look like lotuses.

ACKNOWLEDGMENTS

So many people across the world helped me with my research for this book that I can't begin to list them all. I'm particularly grateful to Agnese Luse, who did invaluable work for me in both Riga and Berlin, and to Nicole Grouman, who helped me conduct interviews in Argentina. Roberto Díaz Herrera was generous with both his time and his anecdotes when I met him in Panama City, as was Piero during our meetings in Argentina. Paul O'Brien was full of colorful stories, told with a wonderfully wry sense of humor. The late B. K. S. Iyengar, a man with endless demands on his time, had the immense kindness to meet with me and share his memories of Krishnamacharya's yoga *shala* when I showed up unannounced at his yoga center in Pune. My friend Anna Pomykala helped me decipher a Polish-language biography of Fryderyk Járosy, and my friends Jessica Heyman and Shirley Velasquez did their best to correct my Spanish in many of my e-mail exchanges. I've learned so much about yoga practice from Lesley Desaulniers and my other wonderful teachers at Prema.

I'm hugely thankful to Lexy Bloom, my meticulous and patient editor at Knopf, as well as to Jenna Dolan, my heroically precise copyeditor. My fact-checkers, Kyla Jones and Ben Phelan, saved me from some truly mortifying mistakes. (Those that may remain are, of course, my responsibility.) This book wouldn't exist without Larry Weissman, my friend and agent. For years, he listened to me say that someone really should write a book about Indra Devi before helping me realize that that person could be me.

When I began researching this book, I had no children. As I finish it, I have two. I couldn't have completed this book while having babies and working in journalism without the support of my husband, Matt Ipcar. I'm thankful to him for so much, from taking me to India so many years ago to accompanying me to Panama with a nursing infant in tow and now reading to our toddler in the next room while I type these acknowledgments. Every blessing in my life begins with him.

NOTES

This book is the product of archival and library research as well as firsthand reporting. Several sources were interviewed multiple times. Direct quotations that come from written sources and from author interviews are indicated in the notes.

INTRODUCTION

3 "As our home industry expands": Gita Mehta, *Karma Cola* (New Delhi, India: Penguin Books India, 1990), p. 7.

5 I ended up writing a story: Michelle Goldberg, "Untouchable?" *Salon*, July 25, 2001, http://www.salon.com/2001/07/25/baba/, accessed September 12, 2014.

7 "what was thought to be the first yoga class": Douglas Martin, "Indra Devi, 102, Dies: Taught Yoga to Stars and Leaders," *New York Times*, April 30, 2002.

10 This opinion is reductive: George Orwell, "Reflections on Gandhi," *Partisan Review*, January 1949.

CHAPTER 1

13 "As a child": Indra Devi, *Una mujer de tres siglos* (Buenos Aires: Editorial Sudamericana, 2000), p. 37.

14 she and her mother had the opportunity to connect: Ibid., p. 67.

14 At the time, Eugenia was already: Natalia Apostolli, *Indra Devi: Una vida, un siglo* (Buenos Aires: Javier Vergara Editor, 1992), p. 22.

14 The building is still standing: Interview with Vladimir Eichenbaums, Riga historian, March 2010.

15 To Eugenia, it seemed: Devi, *Una mujer de tres siglos*, p. 30.

15 There was a constant stream of guests: Ibid., p. 31.

16 "going totally against the conventions of the epoch": Ibid., p. 36.

16 "décolleté"; "coquettish gestures": Yug, review of *Polish Blood*, in *Segodna*, March 20, 1924, p. 5; Yug, review of *Les cloches de Corneville*, in *Segodna*, April 11, 1924.

17 There she insisted: Apostolli, *Indra Devi*, p. 26.

17   For an aristocratic only child: Devi, *Una mujer de tres siglos*, p. 33.

18 Walking beside Sasha: Ibid., p. 39.

19 "We are preparing a little text-book": Yogi Ramacharaka, *Fourteen Lessons in Yogi Philosophy and Oriental Occultism* (Whitefish, MT: Kessinger Publishing, 2003), p. 17.

19 "You are too emotional": Devi, *Una mujer de tres siglos*, p. 40.

19 "Swing back the hands": Yogi Ramacharaka, quoted in Catherine L. Albanese, *A Republic of Mind and Spirit: A Cultural History of American Metaphysical Religion* (New Haven, CT: Yale University Press, 2007), p. 361.

20 "The shelves of the Russian philosophical bookshops": Sir Paul Dukes, *The Yoga of Health, Youth, and Joy* (London: Cassell and Co. Ltd., 1960), p. 5.

20 Between 1881 and 1918: Maria Carlson, *No Religion Higher Than Truth: A History of the Theosophical Movement in Russia, 1875–1922* (Princeton, NJ: Princeton University Press, 1993), p. 21.

20 The work of Papus: Gary Lachman, *Politics and the Occult: The Left, the Right, and the Radically Unseen* (Wheaton, IL: Quest Books, 2008), p. 163.

21 "She may or may not": Peter Washington, *Madame Blavatsky's Baboon: A History of the Mystics, Mediums, and Misfits Who Brought Spiritualism to America* (New York: Schocken Books, 1995), p. 31.

22 "I dwelt upon": Daniel Caldwell, ed., *The Esoteric World of Madame Blavatsky* (Wheaton, IL: Quest Books, 2000), p. 71.

23 "the Folly of Science": Washington, *Madame Blavatsky's Baboon*, p. 45.

23 Her grandfather was the Russian government's administrator: K. Paul Johnson, *The Masters Revealed: Madame Blavatsky and the Myth of the Great White Lodge* (Albany: State University of New York Press, 1994), p. 19.

24 "They were reversing the usual flow of emigration": Washington, *Madame Blavatsky's Baboon*, p. 59.

24 "had many followers in her native land": Sir Paul Dukes, *The Unending Quest: Autobiographical Sketches* (London: Cassell and Co. Ltd., 1950), p. 49.

24 "The people at once had accepted her": Indra Devi, *Forever Young, Forever Healthy: Simplified Yoga for Modern Living* (New York: Prentice Hall, 1953), p. 3.

25 He taught Dukes breathing: Dukes, *The Unending Quest*, p. 106.

25 "For the ignorant, life is delusion": Quoted in R. H. Stacey, *India in Russian Literature* (New Delhi, India: Motilal Banarsidass, 1985), p. 68.

CHAPTER 2

26 Eugenia longed to follow her adored mother: Francesca Falcone and Patrizia Veroli, "The Teaching of Victor Gsovsky in Berlin, 1926–1936, As Seen by Lilian Karina," *Dance Chronicle* 24, no. 3 (2001): 307–50.

26 "Everyone was affected": Richard Pipes, *The Russian Revolution* (New York: Alfred A. Knopf, 1990), p. 237.

27 "We do not take defeat amiss": Quoted in Orlando Figes, *A People's Tragedy: The Russian Revolution 1891–1924* (London: Jonathan Cape, 1996), p. 283.

27 Cafés threw open their doors: Figes, *A People's Tragedy*, pp. 318–19, 351.

27 "A miracle has happened": Ibid., p. 351.

27 Police records were torched: Ibid., p. 317.

27 "All of us who had dreams and projects": Devi, *Una mujer de tres siglos*, p. 46.

28 In March 1917: John E. Malmstad and Nikolaï Alekseevich Bogomolov, *Mikhail Kuzmin: A Life in Art* (Cambridge, MA: Harvard University Press, 1999), pp. 128, 257.

28 Screaming, she feigned panic: Apostolli, *Indra Devi*, p. 32.

28 Her improvisation was, he said: Ibid., p. 32.

29 where she met futurist poets: Ibid., p. 33.

29 "So many horses": Antony Beevor, *The Mystery of Olga Chekhova* (New York: Viking Press, 2004), p. 57.

29 "[m]ost young actresses": Ibid., p. 77.

29 "One morning when a young actress": Theodore Komisarjevsky, *Myself and the Theatre* (London: William Heinemann Ltd., 1929), p. 10.

30 When the guard entered: Apostolli, *Indra Devi*, p. 34.

30 "had an atmosphere of frenzied excitement": Figes, *A People's Tragedy*, p. 555.

31 "All spring": Mikhail Bulgakov, *The White Guard* (New Haven, CT: Yale University Press, 2008), p. 54.

31 He was famous for songs: Richard Sites, *Russian Population Culture: Entertainment and Society Since 1900* (Cambridge, UK: Cambridge University Press, 1995), p. 14.

31 "[e]normous, serene blue": Kohle Yohannan, *Valentina: American Couture and the Cult of Celebrity* (New York: Rizzoli, 2009), p. 26.

31 At his urging: Apostolli, *Indra Devi*, p. 36.

32 Other Chekists devised: Figes, *A People's Tragedy*, p. 646.

32 A touring company: Beevor, *The Mystery of Olga Chekhova*, p. 63.

32 At night, they turned: Devi, *Una mujer de tres siglos*, p. 52.

32 Eugenia, meanwhile: Apostolli, *Indra Devi*, p. 37.

33 "Where did all this come from?": Ibid., p. 35.

33 In a demented inversion: Figes, *A People's Tragedy*, pp. 665, 678.

33 "What brings you here?" . . . "She had learned from her mother": Devi, *Una mujer de tres siglos*, p. 55; Apostolli, *Indra Devi*, p. 40.

34 engraving them in their memories: Devi, *Una mujer de tres siglos*, p. 56.

35 She worried that he had fallen: Ibid., p. 60.

35 More than one hundred thousand Russians: Tom Reiss, *The Orientalist: Solving the Mystery of a Strange and Dangerous Life* (New York: Random House, 2006), pp. 114–15.

36 "Were you in Tiflis?": Devi, *Una mujer de tres siglos, p. 62*; Apostolli, *Indra Devi*, p. 74.

36 On it, she said she'd been held for a month: FBI memo 65-4944, report

made by Roger S. C. Wolcott, obtained through a Freedom of Information Act (FOIA) request; passenger manifest of SS *General William H. Gordon*, NARA microfilm M1410, manifest number 1300-46001, p. EC 18, line 9; private communication with William Greene, Archivist at the National Archives in San Francisco.

37 "I wouldn't do it": Devi, *Una mujer de tres siglos*, pp. 61–64; Apostolli, *Indra Devi*, pp. 74–78.

38 One sounded: Devi, *Una mujer de tres siglos*, p. 66.

38 "Smiling to myself": Ibid., p. 67.

38 She longed to do real theater: Apostolli, *Indra Devi*, pp. 83–84; Devi, *Una mujer de tres siglos*, p. 68.

39 "India appeared to me": Devi, *Una mujer de tres siglos*, p. 68.

CHAPTER 3

40 Berlin's population had doubled: Reiss, *The Orientalist*, p. 171.

40 "After the war": Quoted in John E. Bowlt, "Art in Exile: The Russian Avant-Garde and the Emigration," *Art Journal* 41, no. 3 (Autumn 1981): 215–21.

41 By March of 1923: Bernd Widdig, *Culture and Inflation in Weimar Germany* (Berkeley and Los Angeles: University of California Press, 2001), p. 39.

41 "Herds of foreigners": Quoted in Emil Julius Gumbel, "Four Years of Political Murder," in Anton Kaes, Martin Jay, and Edward Dimendberg, eds., *The Weimar Republic Sourcebook* (Berkeley and Los Angeles: University of California Press, 1994), p. 102.

41 by the mid-1920s: Kaes, Jay, and Dimendberg, eds., *The Weimar Republic Sourcebook*, p. 718; Marlise Simmons, "Amsterdam Tries Upscale Fix for Red Light District Crime," *New York Times*, February 24, 2008.

42 "The indifference with which": Gumbel, "Four Years of Political Murder."

42 "unifies within itself": Kaes, Jay, and Dimendberg, eds., *The Weimar Republic Sourcebook*, p. 554.

42 In her off-hours: Mel Gordon, *Voluptuous Panic: The Erotic World of Weimar Berlin* (Los Angeles: Feral House, 2006), p. ix.

42 An anxious representative: Corinna Treitel, *A Science for the Soul: Occultism and the Creation of the German Modern* (Baltimore and London: Johns Hopkins University Press, 2004), p. 57.

42 Police departments all over: Ibid., p. 144.

43 "and swore on their mezuzahs": Interview with Mel Gordon.

43 "Aspiring occultists": Treitel, *A Science for the Soul*, p. 154.

43 "new, influential metaphysics": Kaes, Jay, and Dimendberg, eds., *The Weimar Republic Sourcebook*, p. 685.

43 As Treitel points out: Treitel, *A Science for the Soul*, p. 25.

44 "[A]gainst every instance": Ibid., p. 160.

44 "The whole thing's lost": Peter Jelavich, *Berlin Cabaret* (Cambridge, MA: Harvard University Press, 1996), p. 143.

44 At once titillating: Alan Lareau, "The German Cabaret Movement during the Weimar Republic," *Theatre Journal* 43, no. 4 (December 1991): 471–90.

45 "pearl of the light genre": Alan Lareau, "Designer Cabaret in 1920s Berlin: The Blue Bird and the Gondola," *Theatre History Studies* 14 (1994).

45 "a world, glowing": Alfred Polgar, quoted in Mark Konecny, ed., *Experiment: A Journal of Russian Culture* 12 (2006).

46 "Der Blaue Vogel": Lareau, "Designer Cabaret in 1920s Berlin," p. 122.

46 "completely in tune with my own": Devi, *Una mujer de tres siglos*, pp. 69–70.

46 "When I met him": Ibid., p. 70.

46 "He was an adventurer": Beevor, *The Mystery of Olga Chekhova*, p. 48.

47 "It was a period": Charles Marowitz, *The Other Chekhov: A Biography of Michael Chekhov, the Legendary Actor, Director, and Theorist* (New York: Applause Theater and Cinema Books, 2004), pp. 70–71.

47 According to her: Beevor, *The Mystery of Olga Chekhova*, p. 77.

47 "eine charmante Frau": Ibid., p. 130.

47 "Tired of politics": Lareau, "Designer Cabaret in 1920s Berlin," pp. 121–22.

48 "[E]verywhere I read": Kaes, Jay, and Dimendberg, eds., *The Weimar Republic Sourcebook*, p. 557.

48 "sublime harmonies": Apostolli, *Indra Devi*, p. 92.

48 Feeling as if she were going crazy: Devi, *Una mujer de tres siglos*, p. 71.

48 Once he arrived: Apostolli, *Indra Devi*, p. 92.

49 "captivated": Interview with Polish theater historian Georgy Suchno, conducted by Agnese Luse. The quote comes from a review by Tadeusz Boy-Żeleński, in Suchno's personal archive.

49 He responded by firing: Devi, *Una mujer de tres siglos*, p. 73.

49 "The only thing that remained": Ibid., p. 73.

49 Indeed, though Eugenia: Ron Nowicki, *Warsaw: The Cabaret Years* (San Francisco: Mercury House, 1992), p. 67.

49 There, she performed: "New Year at A.T.," event listing in *Segodna*, December 30, 1924.

50 He was much changed: Apostolli, *Indra Devi*, p. 96.

50 Suddenly she was shot through with terror: Devi, *Una mujer de tres siglos*, p. 74.

50 She should go to India: Ibid.

50 "All of Warsaw's best": Nowicki, *Warsaw*, p. 50.

50 He intoned: Ibid., p. 67.

51 "The world's leading scholars . . . The epitome of the Nordic race!": Interview with Alicia Nitecki.

52 "A conversation with him": Mieczysław Lurczyński, *The Old Guard: A Play*, trans. (and introduction by) Alicia Nitecki (Albany: Excelsior Editions/State University of New York Press, 2010), p. ix.

52 "Do you know that in": Ibid., p. 21.

52 That's almost certainly: Apostolli, *Indra Devi*, p. 97.

53 With his wavy black hair: Ibid., p. 100.

53 "When we're married": Ibid. p. 101.

54 She wondered if perhaps: Ibid., p. 106.

CHAPTER 4

55 Extra ferries from: Roland Vernon, *Star in the East: Krishnamurti, the Invention of a Messiah* (Boulder, CO: Sentient Publications, 2002), p. 161.

55 "Such readers as have ever": Rom Landau, *God Is My Adventure: A Book on Modern Mystics, Masters, and Teachers* (London: Faber and Faber, 1964), p. 89.

56 "The camp is beautifully situated": Associated Press, "Secrecy Veils Cult Camp," *Los Angeles Times*, July 29, 1926.

56 Attendees carried their own plates: Mary Lutyens, *Krishnamurti: The Years of Awakening* (Boston: Shambala,1997), p. 232.

56 "insipid": Devi, *Una mujer de tres siglos*, p. 79; Devi, *Forever Young, Forever Healthy*, p. 5.

57 "You give me phrases": Lutyens, *Krishnamurti*, p. 233.

57 "Whenever He speaks": A.E.L., "A Spiritual Aristocracy," *Herald of the Star* 15, no. 9, September 1, 1926.

58 Madame Blavatsky and Henry Steele Olcott's: Washington, *Madame Blavatsky's Baboon*, p. 59.

58 "The fundamental appeal": Mark Bevir, "Theosophy and the Origins of the Indian National Congress," *International Journal of Hindu Studies* 7, no. 1/3 (February 2003).

59 "The greatest recent event": Friedrich Nietzsche, *The Gay Science,* ed. Bernard Williams (Cambridge, UK: Cambridge University Press, 2001), p. 343.

59 "In the minds of many Victorians": Bevir, "Theosophy and the Origins of the Indian National Congress."

60 "For our own part": Carlson, *No Religion Higher Than Truth*, p. 42.

60 Under pressure from Olcott: Washington, *Madame Blavatsky's Baboon*, p. 85.

60 "stimulated in me the desire": Mahatma Gandhi, *An Autobiography: The Story of My Experiments with Truth* (Boston: Beacon Press, 1993), p. 68.

61 "Oh, my dear": Arthur Nethercot, *The First Five Lives of Annie Besant* (Chicago: University of Chicago Press, 1960), p. 286.

61 "Mme. Blavatsky": Ibid., p. 199.

61 "Are you willing to give up": Ibid., p. 293.

62 "Staggered by this unprepared blow": Quoted in ibid., p. 283.

63 "Glad sensation": Lutyens, *Krishnamurti*, p. 15.

63 "My dear Annie": Ibid., p. 17.

63 According to his lifelong friend: Ibid., p. 21.

64 "The Brahmins of India": The Reverend W. B. Norton, "Krishnamurti, East Indian, Is Declared Returned Messiah," *Chicago Daily Tribune*, March 29, 1926.

65 "a turning point in my life": Devi, *Forever Young, Forever Healthy*, p. 5.

65 Shortly after she'd come home: Devi, *Una mujer de tres siglos*, pp. 81–82.

66 She kept working in the theater: Apostolli, *Indra Devi*, p. 110.

66 "an Englishwoman of great dignity": G. Venkatachalam, *Profiles* (Baroda, India: Nalanda Publications Co., 1949), p. 299.

66 "It's better that she goes": Apostolli, *Indra Devi*, p. 111.

66 "I was in a state": Devi, *Forever Young, Forever Healthy*, p. 6.

67 "[h]appy beyond measure": Ibid., p. 7.

CHAPTER 5

71 "like an ancient Druid priest": Major-General the Hon. Kenneth Mackay, "Adyar—An Impression," *The Theosophist* 49, part 1 (October 1927–March 1928).

71 Visitors entered: *The Theosophist* 49, part 2 (April–September 1928).

72 Inside the main meeting hall: J. Krishnamurti, with descriptive letterpress by C. W. Leadbeater, *Adyar: The Home of the Theosophical Society* (Adyar, Madras, India: The Theosophist Office, 1911).

72 "Never shake hands": Margaret MacMillan, *Women of the Raj: The Mothers, Wives, and Daughters of the British Empire in India* (New York: Random House, 2007), p. xii.

72 "untrammeled alike": Mackay, "Adyar—An Impression."

72 "Here," writes Mackay, "it has been": Ibid.

73 "artists and art students": Venkatachalam, *Profiles*, p. 299.

73 "Adyar becomes a miniature world": Ibid., p. 40.

73 "with bazaars and restaurants": Ibid.

74 Besant was convinced: Washington, *Madame Blavatsky's Baboon*, p. 257.

74 The attempt to create an organization: Ibid., p. 275.

74 "Out of those who come to listen": N. R. Deobankar, "Krishnaji at Adyar," *The Theosophist* 50, part 1 (October 1928–March 1929).

75 she would compile a list of problems: Indra Devi, *Una mujer de tres siglos*, pp. 85–86.

75 "All humanity's greatest": Krishna Kripalani, *Rabindranath Tagore: A Biography* (Calcutta, India: Visva-Bharati Publishing Department, 1980), p. 305.

76 "Yatra visvam bhavati": Visva-Bharati website, http://www.visvabharati.ac .in/EDUCATIONAL_IDEAS.html, accessed October 18, 2014.

76 "You will find a famous European Scholar": *Visva-Bharati: A Visitor's Impression of Santiketan*, pamphlet distributed by the India Society of America, February 1929.

76 Eugenia adored it: Devi, *Una mujer de tres siglos*, p. 87.

77 "By God's infinite blessing": Quoted in Kumari Jayawardena, *The White Woman's Other Burden: Western Women and South Asia during British Rule* (New York: Routledge, 1995), p. 199.

78 Life in Europe seemed gray: Devi, *Una mujer de tres siglos*, p. 90.

79 "I maintain that Truth is a pathless land": Lutyens, *Krishnamurti*, pp. 272–74.

80 "Thousands felt betrayed": Vernon, *Star in the East*, p. 185.

80 "My fundamental belief": Associated Press, "Mrs. Besant Loyal to Krishnamurti," *New York Times*, August 6, 1929.

81 "Amma says to me"; "get out of all this rot": Lutyens, *Krishnamurti*, p. 277; Vernon, *Star in the East*, p. 185.

81 Traveling cinemas: Priti Ramamurthy, "The Modern Girl in India in the Interwar Years: Interracial Intimacies, International Competition, and Historical Eclipsing," *Women's Studies Quarterly* 34, no. 1/2, The Global and the Intimate (Spring/Summer 2006).

82 Musicians accompanied screenings: Suresh Chabria, ed., *Light of Asia: Indian Silent Cinema, 1912–1934* (New Delhi, India: Wiley Eastern Limited, 1994).

82 "Film Actors": Neepa Majumdar, *Wanted Cultured Ladies Only! Female Stardom and Cinema in India, 1930s–1950s* (Urbana and Chicago: University of Illinois Press, 2009), p. 41.

82 "It is really a perplexing problem": Ganeshiam U. Vaswani, "Social Status of Film Stars," *Cinema*, June–July 1931.

82 After the smashing success: Ramamurthy, "The Modern Girl in India in the Interwar Years"; Majumdar, *Wanted Cultured Ladies Only!*, p. 95.

83 "God, I have come": Madhu Jain, *The Kapoors: The First Family of Indian Cinema* (New Delhi, India: Viking/Penguin Books India, 2005), p. 3.

83 "The Nehru-Gandhis": Ibid., p. xvi.

83 She told Mishra: Apostolli, *Indra Devi*, p. 129.

CHAPTER 6

84 "Jean is an artist of a sort": Venkatachalam, *Profiles*, p. 308.

85 His salary was just enough: Apostolli, *Indra Devi*, p. 131; Jain, *The Kapoors*, p. 10.

85 "excellent force: Jan Strakaty personal service record, electronic file sent to the author by the Czech Foreign Ministry Archives, Prague.

85 Instead, he went: Apostolli, *Indra Devi*, p. 134.

86 In the end: Devi, *Una mujer de tres siglos*, p. 97; Apostolli, Indra Devi, p. 135.

86 "in that manner": Devi, *Una mujer de tres siglos*, p. 97.

87 "Don't try": MacMillan, *Women of the Raj*, p. 48.

87 One friend even warned her: Apostolli, *Indra Devi*, p. 140.

87 A friend of hers: Devi, *Una mujer de tres siglos*, p. 97.

88 "Her rooms": Venkatachalam, *Profiles*, p. 168.

88 "our Mickey Mouse": Vishwanath S. Naravane, *Sarojini Nairu: Her Life, Work, and Poetry* (Hyderabad, India: Orient Longman Limited, 1996), p. 149.

88 "Akka": Apostolli, *Indra Devi*, p. 142.

88 Sure enough: Naravane, *Sarojini Naidu*, pp. 62, 149.

89 "The young ones among": Shashi Tharoor, *Nehru: The Invention of India* (New York: Arcade Publishing, 2003), p. 71.

89 "The object of jail": Stanley Wolpert, *Nehru: A Tryst with Destiny* (New York: Oxford University Press, 1996), p. 113.

90 "It's a complete reversal": Frank Moraes, *Jawaharlal Nehru: A Biography* (Mumbai, India: Jaico Publishing House, 2008), p. 221.

90 "This old and typical": Jawaharlal Nehru, *The Discovery of India* (New Delhi, India: Oxford University Press, 1985), p. 186.

90 "As you seemed to be interested": Nehru letter to Devi, provided by the Fundación Indra Devi, Buenos Aires, Argentina.

90 "Certainly I would like": Ibid.

91 "I felt that I was being initiated": Devi, *Una mujer de tres siglos*, p. 104.

91 "Was this why I had come": Devi, *Forever Young, Forever Healthy*, pp. 9–10.

92 "passes his hand": Yogi Ramacharaka, *Fourteen Lessons in Yogi Philosophy* (New York: Cosimo Inc., 2007), p. 148.

93 "Less energetic women": MacMillan, *Women of the Raj*, p. 102.

94 "The next morning I woke up": Devi, *Forever Young, Forever Healthy*, p. 14.

CHAPTER 7

95 "No respectable people": " 'Sadhus' on the Chowpatty Foreshore," *Times of India*, September 15, 1932.

95 "through the rows of mushroom-like umbrellas": Eugenie Strakaty (Indira Devi), *Yoga: The Technique of Health and Happiness* (Allahabad, India: Kitabistan, 1948), p. 18.

96 The men were naked or nearly: Devi, *Forever Young, Forever Healthy*, p. 1.

96 "But these are not yogis": Ibid., p. 2.

96 "torture and self-maceration": H. P. Blavatsky, *The Secret Doctrine: The Synthesis of Science, Religion, and Philosophy, Volume 1: Cosmogenesis* (London: The Theosophical Publishing Society, 1893), p. 78.

96 "We have nothing": Swami Vivekananda, *Raja Yoga* (New York: Ramakrishna-Vivekananda Center, 1982), p. 23.

97 "the word *yoga*": Mircea Eliade, *Yoga: Immortality and Freedom* (Princeton, NJ: Princeton University Press, 2009), p. 4.

97 "The posture": Georg Feuerstein, *The Yoga-Sutra of Pantanjali: A New Translation and Commentary* (Rochester, VT: Inner Traditions International, 1989), p. 154

98 "Yoga is the restriction": Ibid., p. 26.

98 "Depend upon it": Quoted in J. J. Clarke, *Oriental Enlightenment: The Encounter between Eastern and Western Thought* (New York: Routledge, 2003), p. 87.

98 "one of the greatest things": Ibid., p. 155.

99 "presupposes that we turn": Feuerstein, *The Yoga-Sutra of Pantanjali*, pp. 10–11.

99 "the term": Eliade, *Yoga: Immortality and Freedom*, p. 35.

99 The first of these books: Ibid., p. 230; James Mallinson, *The Shiva Sam-*

hita: A Critical Edition and English Translation (Woodstock, NY: YogaVidya, 2007), pp. 63–70.

100 "worship of the goddess": Wendy Doniger, *The Hindus: An Alternative History* (New York: Penguin Press, 2009), p. 419.

100 "Five Jewels": Ibid., p. 424.

100 "the function of an organ": Arthur Koestler, *The Lotus and the Robot* (New York: Macmillan, 1961), pp. 130–31.

100 "The Yogi who can protect": *The Hatha Yoga Pradipika*, trans. Pancham Singh, e-book (no publisher, 1915), n.p.

100 "must be blocked": Koestler, *The Lotus and the Robot*, pp. 130–31.

100 "He who knows": *The Hatha Yoga Pradipika*, trans. Pancham Singh, e-book (no publisher, 1915), n.p.

101 "Subtle physiology": Eliade, *Yoga: Immortality and Freedom*, pp. 233–34.

101 "Jauguis": Mark Singleton, *Yoga Body: The Origins of Modern Posture Practice* (New York: Oxford University Press, 2010), p. 37.

102 "highly organized bands": Ibid., p. 39.

102 According to G. S. Ghurye: G. S. Ghurye, *Indian Sadhus* (Bombay, India: Popular Prakashan, 1964), p. 112.

102 "almost the counterpart": Singleton, *Yoga Body*, p. 41.

102 "explain the apparent discrepancy": Ibid.

102 "No longer able": Ibid., p. 40.

103 "Religion, like the white light": Quoted in Rev. John Henry Barrows, ed., *The World's Parliament of Religions: An Illustrated and Popular Story of the World's First Parliament of Religions, Held in Chicago in Connection with the Columbian Exposition of 1893* (Chicago: Parliament Publishing Co., 1893), p. 3.

103 Mary Baker Eddy: Albanese, *A Republic of Mind and Spirit*, p. 333.

103 Many attendees were Theosophists: Ibid., p. 332.

104 "clad in gorgeous red apparel": Barrows, *The World's Parliament of Religions*, p. 62.

104 "disgusted": Vikram Sampath, *Splendours of Royal Mysore: The Untold Story of the Wodeyars* (New Delhi, India: Rupa and Co., 2009), p. 514.

104 "By preaching": Narasingha P. Sil, "Vivekānanda's Rāmakṛṣṇa: An Untold Story of Mythmaking and Propaganda," *Numen* 40, no. 1 (January 1993).

105 "As our country": Quoted in Elizabeth De Michelis, *A History of Modern Yoga* (London: Continuum, 2005), p. 109.

105 "Allow me": Harold W. French, *The Swan's White Way: Ramakrishna and Western Culture* (Port Washington, NY: Kennikat Press, 1974), p. 57.

105 "undoubtedly the greatest": Ibid., p. 55.

105 When his book *Raja Yoga*: Albanese, *A Republic of Mind and Spirit*, p. 354.

105 Schwartz argues: Evan I. Schwartz, *Finding Oz: How L. Frank Baum Discovered the Great American Story* (New York: Houghton Mifflin Harcourt, 2009), p. 276.

106 "Sandow looks and feels": Mark Adams, *Mr. America: How Muscular Mil-*

lionaire Bernarr Macfadden Transformed the Nation through Sex, Salad, and the Ultimate Starvation Diet (New York: Harper, 2009), p. 34; "He Is a Man of Mighty Muscle," *Chicago Tribune*, August 11, 1893.

106 "Behold the mighty Englishman": Gandhi, *An Autobiography*, p. 21.

107 "The entire country": Narasingha Prosad Sil, *Swami Vivekananda: A Reassessment* (Cranbury, NJ: Associated University Presses, 1997), p. 53.

107 "How will you struggle": Singleton, *Yoga Body*, p. 100.

107 "electrified": "Sandow's Visit to Bombay," *Times of India*, November 23, 1904.

107 Local newspapers heaped: David L. Chapman, *Sandow the Magnificent: Eugen Sandow and the Beginnings of Bodybuilding* (Urbana and Chicago: University of Illinois Press, 1994), pp. 157–58.

107 The Maharaja of Baroda: Michael Anton Budd, *The Sculpture Machine: Physical Culture and Body Politics in the Age of Empire* (New York: New York University Press, 1997), p. 84.

107 "The native Indians": Quoted in Chapman, *Sandow the Magnificent*, p. 157.

108 "He reminded me": Koestler, *The Lotus and the Robot*, p. 102.

108 "He opened out": Joseph Alter, *Yoga in Modern India: The Body between Science and Philosophy* (Princeton, NJ: Princeton University Press, 2004), p. 81.

108 He read the works: Alter, *Yoga in Modern India*, p. 82; Alter, "*Gandhi's Body*, p. 67.

109 To Gandhi, for example: Mandhar Gharote and Manmath Gharote, *Swami Kuvalayananda: A Pioneer of Scientific Yoga and Indian Physical Education* (Lonavla, India: Lonavla Yoga Institute, 1999), p. 97.

109 There, he began: "Yogic Exercises for Women," *Times of India* (1861); April 27, 1935.

110 "Which will probably be": Devi, *Forever Young, Forever Healthy*, p. 17.

110 Certainly, as she spent: Apostolli, *Indra Devi*, pp. 167–68.

111 Seeking to escape the tedious social whirl: Ibid., p. 169.

CHAPTER 8

112 Gandhi called the Maharaja: Sampath, *Splendours of Royal Mysore*, p. 521.

112 The maharaja built universities: James Manor, *Political Change in an Indian State: Mysore 1917–1955* (Columbia, MO: South Asia Books, 1978), p. 12.

113 The maharaja was: Sampath, *Splendours of Royal Mysore*, p. 649.

113 "absorbed the best": Annie Cahn Fung, "Paul Brunton: A Bridge between India and the West," translated from "Paul Brunton: un pont entre l'Inde et l'Occident," doctoral thesis, Department of Religious Anthropology, Université de Paris IV, Sorbonne, 1992, p. 57.

113 "a pan-Indian hub": Singleton, *Yoga Body*, p. 100.

114 A manual compiled: See N. E. Sjoman, *The Yoga Tradition of the Mysore Palace* (New Delhi, India: Abhinav Publications, 1999).

115 "You may have never": Fernando Pagés Ruiz, "Krishnamacharya's Legacy," *Yoga Journal*, May/June 2001.

115 Upon awakening: Kausthub Desikachar, *The Yoga of the Yogi: The Legacy of T. Krishnamacharya* (Chennai, India: Krishnamacharya Yoga Mandiram, 2005), pp. 31–33.

116 Krishnamacharya claimed that: Pagés Ruiz, "Krishnamacharya's Legacy."

116 At the end: Desikachar, *The Yoga of the Yogi*, pp. 54–60.

116 On his days off: Pagés Ruiz, "Krishnamacharya's Legacy."

117 They concluded that: M. A. Wenger, B. K. Bagchi, and B. K. Anand, "Experiments in India on 'Voluntary' Control of the Heart and Pulse," *Circulation* 24 (1961).

117 "The Physical Instruction": Singleton, *Yoga Body*, p. 179.

118 As Singleton has shown: Ibid., pp. 199–201.

118 From there, the practitioner: Ibid., p. 200.

118 "It is quite clear": Sjoman, *The Yoga Tradition of the Mysore Palace*, pp. 53–55.

119 *Life* magazine sent a photographer: "Heir to $400,000,000 Gets Married in India," *Life*, August 15, 1938.

119 Festivities began with: "200 Prisoners Set Free: Mysore Ruler's Clemency," *Times of India*, May 16, 1938.

119 "presented a scene": Ibid.

119 "In my school there are no women": Kausthub Desikachar, *The Yoga of the Yogi: The Legacy of T. Krishnamacharya* (Chennai, India: Krishnamacharya Yoga Mandiram, 2005), p. 99.

120 Eugenia tried to: Apostolli, *Indra Devi*, p. 171.

120 "Guruji had a frightful personality": B. K. S. Iyengar, *Astadala Yogamala: Collected Works*, vol. 1 (Mumbai, India: Allied Publishers Private Ltd., 2000), p. 52.

120 "My sisters and sisters-in-law": Ibid., p. 22.

121 "Why are you going to complicate": Devi, *Una mujer de tres siglos*, p. 115.

121 "From now on": Strakaty, *Yoga: The Technique of Health and Happiness*, p. 30.

122 "I imagined": Ibid., p. 31.

122 "The European student": Devi, *Una mujer de tres siglos*, p. 117.

123 This notion that yoga: P. Singh et al., "The Impact of Yoga upon Female Patients Suffering from Hypothyroidism," *Complementary Therapies in Clinical Practice* (2010), doi:10.1016/j.ctcp.2010.11.004; Beth E. Cohen, et al., "Feasibility and Acceptability of Restorative Yoga for Treatment of Hot Flushes: A Pilot Trial," *Maturitas* 56, no. 2 (February 20, 2007); Suresh C. Jain et al., "A Study of Response Pattern of Non-Insulin Dependent Diabetics to Yoga Therapy," *Diabetes Research and Clinical Practice*, 19, no. 1 (January 1993).

123 "interact reciprocally": Paul Salmon et al., "Yoga and Mindfulness: Clinical Aspects of an Ancient Mind/Body Practice," *Cognitive and Behavioral Practice* 16, no. 1 (February 2009).

123 "I felt as light": Devi, *Forever Young, Forever Healthy*, p. 19.

124 "He told her that": Ibid., p. 21.

124 "Now that you are going to visit": Apostolli, *Indra Devi*, p. 175.

CHAPTER 9

127 Encountering her new home: Devi, *Una mujer de tres siglos*, p. 119.

127 "far advanced along the spiritual path": Audrey Youngman, "The Grande Dame of Yoga," *Yoga Journal*, October 1996.

128 "I understood then why": Strakaty, *Yoga: The Technique of Health and Happiness*, p. 58.

128 "Do you know": Youngman, "The Grande Dame of Yoga."

128 "I discovered that I didn't": Strakaty, *Yoga: The Technique of Health and Happiness*, pp. 62–63.

129 "As you stepped ashore": Harriet Sergeant, *Shanghai* (London: John Murray, 1999), p. 3.

129 Thousands of Eastern European: Horst "Peter" Eisfelder, *Chinese Exile: My Years in Shanghai and Nanking* (Bergenfield, NJ: Avotaynu Foundation, 2003), p. 39.

130 The White Russians: Sergeant, *Shanghai*, p. 31.

130 There were six daily: Marcia Reynders Ristaino, *Port of Last Resort: The Diaspora Communities of Shanghai* (Stanford, CA: Stanford University Press, 2001), p. 84.

130 "everything from handbags": Emily Hahn, *China to Me*, E-reads reprint, 1999, p. 81.

131 The occupiers waged a terror: Stella Dong, *Shanghai: The Rise and Fall of a Decadent City* (New York: HarperPerennial, 2001), p. 264; John B. Powell, *My Twenty-Five Years in China*, full text available at http://archive.org /stream/mytwentyfiveyear009218mbp/mytwentyfiveyear009218mbp_djvu .txt.

131 "Do anything you want": Strakaty, *Yoga: The Technique of Health and Happiness*, pp. 63, 70.

132 Yet, instead of quitting: Jan Strakaty personal service record, electronic file obtained from the Czech Ministry of Foreign Affairs, Prague.

132 Jan had kept his Czech passport: Ibid.; "Baltic Citizens in China Offered Soviet Citizenship," *China Weekly Review*, September 28, 1940.

132 "The members of the 'Circle'": Jan Strakaty personal service record.

133 "without prior notification": Ibid.

133 He and Jan Seba tried: Ibid.

133 The first person to call: Devi, *Una mujer de tres siglos*, p. 121.

133 Then someone suggested: Strakaty, *Yoga: The Technique of Health and Happiness*, pp. 64–70.

134 By day, Devi turned: Ibid., p. 71.

134 "We did the exercises": Youngman, "The Grande Dame of Yoga."

134 "Before we start" . . . "In the more advanced stages": Strakaty, *Yoga: The*

Technique of Health and Happiness, pp. 91–113; Indra Devi, *Yoga for Americans: An Authentic Course for Home Practice* (MACE Records, exact date unknown).

136 "Mrs. B.": Strakaty, *Yoga: The Technique of Health and Happiness*, p. 23.

136 The American military attaché: FBI report made by Woodrow P. Lipscomb, September 15, 1950, obtained through FOIA request.

136 "I don't know anything": Hahn, *China to Me*, p. 82.

137 He gave her a shiny blue: Ken Cuthbertson, *Nobody Said Not to Go: The Life, Loves, and Adventures of Emily Hahn* (Boston: Faber and Faber, 1998), p. 135.

137 "She was an eccentric person": Hahn, *China to Me*, p. 82.

137 "Sorry we cannot extend": Ibid., p. 107.

138 "shaking her head": Ibid., p. 82.

138 These days of silence drove: Strakaty, *Yoga: The Technique of Health and Happiness*, p. 84.

138 "Sinmay adored her": Hahn, *China to Me*, p. 82.

138 "I was spending": Ibid.

138 "Mr. Levin's image" . . . So she withdrew: Ibid., p. 83.

138 "Probably in the back": Ibid., p. 108.

139 "Zhenia!": Apostolli, *Indra Devi*, p. 192.

139 Avshalomov fell in love: Jacob Avshalomov and Aaron Avshalomov, *Avshalomov's Winding Way: Composers Out of China—A Chronicle* (Bloomington, IN: Xlibris, 2002), p. 37.

140 He found increasing success: Avshalomov and Avshalomov, *Avshalomov's Winding Way*, p. 65.

140 "I feel old and tired": Ibid., p. 148.

140 "rehearsing the Indian": Ibid., p. 151.

141 "Indira Devi danced": Ibid., p. 152.

141 "Creative work": Ibid., p. 163.

141 "kindred souls": Report by William G. Osborn of interview with Mrs. H. H. Vreeland, FBI file 65-1804, obtained through FOIA request.

141 "The ballet has": Avshalomov and Avshalomov, *Avshalomov's Winding Way*, p. 167.

141 "To get into a movie": Vanya Oakes, *White Man's Folly* (Boston: Houghton Mifflin Co., 1943), p. 357.

141 "Shanghai": Ibid., p. 359.

142 "There on the river stretch": Edna Lee Booker, *Flight from China* (New York: Macmillan Co., 1945), p. 131.

142 "The Imperial Japanese": Ibid., p. 133

143 "I shall never forget": Strakaty, *Yoga: The Technique of Health and Happiness*, pp. 68–69.

143 "with a Japanese sentry": Ibid., p. 69.

143 Years later: Youngman "The Grande Dame of Yoga."

143 "Stood for 1½ hours": Peggy Abkhazi, *The Curious Cage: A Shanghai Journal 1941–1945* (Victoria, BC: Sono Nis Press, 1981), p. 22.

143 "We could hardly": Booker, *Flight from China*, p. 133.

144 The red armbands: Ibid., p. 153.

144 The Japanese froze: Stella Dong, *Shanghai: The Rise and Fall of a Decadent City* (New York: HarperPerennial, 2001), p. 270.

144 Those who could afford: Booker, *Flight from China*, p. 151.

144 "Hundreds of Chinese": Ibid., p. 150.

144 "The Russian community": Ristaino, *Port of Last Resort*, p. 237.

144 After the war: Youngman, "The Grande Dame of Yoga," p. 78.

145 She continued giving: Ibid.

145 "On certain days": Dong, *Shanghai*, p. 277.

146 Some industrious camp inmates: Strakaty, *Yoga: The Technique of Health and Happiness*, p. 68.

146 Eventually, when a Japanese: Devi, *Una mujer de tres siglos*, p 125.

146 "it was almost": Valentin V. Fedoulenko, "Russian Émigré Life in Shanghai," interview conducted by Boris Raymond in July, August, and September 1966, published by the University of California, Bancroft Library/Berkeley Regional Oral History Office, 1967. Full text available at http://archive.org/stream/russianemigrbeshanoofedorich/russianemigrbeshanoofedorich_djvu.txt.

146 "to be either": Youngman, "The Grande Dame of Yoga."

147 One day, she told Jan: Apostolli, *Indra Devi*, p. 195–96.

147 "new and most cruel bomb." Emperor Hirohito, accepting the Potsdam Declaration, Radio Broadcast, transmitted by Domei and recorded by the Federal Communications Commission, August 14, 1945, transcript available at https://www.mtholyoke.edu/acad/intrel/hirohito.htm.

147 "Wherever we went": Ristaino, *Port of Last Resort*, p. 243.

147 "Shanghai is now": Avshalomov and Avshalomov, *Avshalomov's Winding Way*, p. 202.

148 "I was interested"; "Indira Devi's much-advertised": K. P. S. Menon, *Twilight in China* (Bombay, India: Bharatiya Vidya Bhavan, 1972), pp. 125, 135.

148 "I firmly believe": Avshalomov and Avshalomov, *Avshalomov's Winding Way*, p. 226.

148 A few months later: Jan Strakaty personal service record.

CHAPTER 10

150 "the paradise of hermits": Mircea Eliade, *Autobiography, Volume 1: 1907–1937* (Chicago: University of Chicago Press, 1981), p. 188.

150 "well-regulated diet": Sarah Strauss, "Adapt, Adjust, Accommodate: The Production of Yoga in a Transnational World," in Mark Singleton and Jean Byrne, eds., *Yoga in the Modern World: Contemporary Perspectives*, e-book (London and New York: Routledge, 2008), n.p.

150 "His approach to solving": Ibid.

150 "an ideal place": Ibid.

151 like a dog grateful for scraps: Devi, *Una mujer de tres siglos*, p. 129.

151 "Come tomorrow and study": Apostolli, *Indra Devi*, p. 205.

151 Like Vivekananda: Sarah Strauss, *Positioning Yoga* (Oxford, UK: Berg, 2005), p. 9.

151 Back at the castle: Devi, *Una mujer de tres siglos*, p. 129.

151 At times: Devi, *Forever Young, Forever Healthy*, p. 11.

152 "[g]rief, mental distress": Vivekananda, *Raja Yoga*, p. 126.

152 Her teacher told her: Apostolli, *Indra Devi*, p. 207.

152 "People are coming": Strakaty, *Yoga: The Technique of Health and Happiness*, p. 51.

152 "blindly copying the West": Ibid., p. 89.

153 Bhante's ideas about healing: Barbara Stewart, "Bellong Mahathera Is Dead; Cambodian Monk was 110," *New York Times*, July 18, 1999; Michael York, *Historical Dictionary of New Age Movements* (Lanham, MD: Scarecrow Press, 2004), p. 60.

153 While in the city: Program for *The Great Wall*, presented by the China Welfare Fund Committee, and in the author's possession.

154 "[T]hose who have seen": Quoted in the program for *Aaron Avshalomov: New Expression to Chinese Music and Theater*, in author's possession.

CHAPTER 11

156 "no woman shall": "Palatial Home Is Finished," *Los Angeles Times*, November 15, 1914.

157 She had six thousand dollars: Report by Roger S. C. Wolcott, FBI File 65-4944, obtained through FOIA request.

157 "The only thing left to do": Devi, *Una mujer de tres siglos*, p. 133.

158 "I try to live in the eternal now": Interview with David Lifar.

159 "Aldous Huxley": David King Dunway, *Huxley in Hollywood* (New York: Anchor Books, 1991), p. 14.

159 "when they are not": William Tindall, "The Trouble with Aldous Huxley," *The American Scholar* 11, no. 4 (Autumn 1942).

160 "The ideal man": Strakaty, *Yoga: The Technique of Health and Happiness*, p. 60.

160 All that she recorded: Devi, *Forever Young, Forever Healthy*, pp. 52–53.

160 "How can you expect": Aldous Huxley, *Eyeless in Gaza* (New York: Harper Perennial, 1995), pp. 422–24.

161 "a mind reader": Robert Love, *The Great Oom: The Improbable Birth of Yoga in America* (New York: Viking, 2010), p. 12.

161 "advanced physical culture": Ibid., p. 13.

161 Bernard first used his skills: Ibid., p. 20.

161 "a band of dashing gypsy": Ibid., p. 30.

161 "'Hindoo Priest' Lures Girls": *Chicago Daily Tribune*, May 4, 1910.

161 "Wild Orgies": "Wild Orgies in the Temple of 'Om,'" *San Francisco Chronicle*, May 5, 1910.

161 "Coroner Holds 'Hindu Yogi'": *New York Tribune*, June 19, 1910.

162 "the Hindu with the": "Massaging Too Much for Her: Woman Causes Hindu Hypnotist's Downfall," *Los Angeles Times*, May 14, 1910.

162 "A Hindu Apple": "A Hindu Apple for the Modern Eve," *Los Angeles Times*, October 22, 1911.

162 Unlike most other tabloid: Love, *The Great Oom*, p. 113.

162 "Lawyers and teachers": Ibid., p. 114.

162 In 1920 he set up: Catherine Albanese, "Sacred (and Secular) Self-Fashioning: Esalen and the American Transformation of Yoga," in Jeffrey John Kripal and Glenn W. Shuck, eds., *On the Edge of the Future: Esalen and the Transformation of American Culture* (Bloomington: Indiana University Press, 2005), p. 65.

162 "Mahatma": Edith Wharton, *Twilight Sleep* (New York: Scribner, 1997), p. 23.

163 Indeed, when Devi gave: Devi, *Forever Young, Forever Healthy*, p. 23.

164 It's not clear if: Avshalomov and Avshalomov, *Avshalomov's Winding Way*, p. 275.

164 He was not, however: Ibid., p. 291.

164 for which she received $4,500: Report by Roger S. Wolcott, Los Angeles, July 3, 1950, FBI File 65-4944, obtained through FOIA request.

164 "[P]robably when I am": Avshalomov and Avshalomov, *Avshalomov's Winding Way*, p. 277.

164 "I felt that underlying": Ibid., p. 295.

164 "No matter what I do": Ibid., p. 296.

165 "Before this war": Report from Shanghai, China, April 20, 1948, National Archives.

165 "philosophical concepts of yoga": Report by Mr. D. L. Nicholson to J. Edgar Hoover, October 19, 1950, obtained through FOIA request.

165 Colonel M. B. DePass: Report by Woodrow P. Lipscomb, September 15, 1950, FBI File 65-1671, obtained through FOIA request.

165 "sufficiently intelligent": Report by Roger S. C. Wolcott, July 31, 1950, FBI File 65-4944, obtained through FOIA request.

165 "In view of the original allegations": Memo from the FBI director to SAC, Los Angeles, March 16, 1950, FBI File 65-58839-8, obtained through FOIA request.

166 Being under investigation: Report by Roger S. C. Wolcott, July 31, 1950, FBI File 65-4944, obtained through FOIA request.

CHAPTER 12

167 "sumptuous starvation": "Billions of Dollars for Prettiness: Big Industry Thrives on Woman's Struggle to Stay Young," *Life*, December 24, 1956.

168 After a stint in Arizona: Report by Roger S. C. Wolcott, July 31, 1950, FBI file 65-4944, obtained through FOIA request.

168 "The two women would": Kohle Yohannan, *Valentina: American Couture and the Cult of Celebrity* (New York: Rizzoli, 2009), p. 160.

169 "standing on her head": Christopher Challis, *Are They Really So Awful? A Cameraman's Chronicles* (London: Janus Publishing Co., 1995), p. 89.

169 "During one yoga lesson": Marion Mill Preminger, *All I Want Is Everything* (New York: Funk and Wagnalls Co., 1957), p. 178.

169 "had taken on": Robert Balzer, *Beyond Conflict* (Indianapolis: Bobbs-Merrill Co., 1963), p. 170.

170 The film made use: Sam Kashner and Jennifer MacNair, *The Bad and the Beautiful: Hollywood in the Fifties* (New York: W. W. Norton, 2002), p. 337.

170 "that were awful imitations": Gloria Swanson, *Swanson on Swanson* (New York: Pocket Books, 1980), p. 506.

170 In 1976: Kashner and MacNair, *The Bad and the Beautiful*, p. 347.

171 how to sleep better: Devi, *Forever Young, Forever Healthy*," p. 25.

171 "I shall not": Ibid., p. 31.

171 "about someone's 'uncle' ": Ibid., p. 64.

171 "Your hips perhaps?": Ibid., p. 118.

172 By today's standards: Ibid., p. 119.

172 "by the route of male achievement": Marynia Farnham and Ferdinand Lundberg book quoted in Betty Friedan, *The Feminine Mystique* (New York: W. W. Norton, 2001), pp. 119–20.

172 "It is a well known fact": Devi, *Forever Young, Forever Healthy*, p. 107.

172 "very important": Ibid., p. 111.

173 "more beautifully": Ibid., p. 116.

173 At the last minute: Letter from Gloria Swanson to Indra Devi, June 6, 1953, Gloria Swanson Papers, Harry Ransom Humanities Research Center, University of Texas at Austin.

173 "Gloria Swanson's latest": Walter Winchell, "Of New York," *Washington Post*, November 25, 1953.

173 "Among the 'sideline' ": Aline Mosby, "Hollywood Yoga Teacher Puts Stars through Paces," *Spokane Chronicle*, January 2, 1954.

174 "What are you doing?": Jack Zaiman, "The Needle's Eye: They Call Me Yoga," *Hartford Courant*, October 27, 1953.

174 Swanson cabled Devi: Telegraph from Swanson to Devi, February 15, 1954, Gloria Swanson Papers, Harry Ransom Humanities Research Center, University of Texas at Austin.

174 At the end of a four-page letter to Swanson: Letter from Indra Devi to Gloria Swanson, August 14 (year not given), Gloria Swanson Papers, Harry Ransom Humanities Research Center, University of Texas at Austin.

CHAPTER 13

175 In her autobiography: Devi, *Una mujer de tres siglos*, p. 136; Letter from Sigfrid Knauer to the House of Representatives, April 4, 1956, *United States Congressional Serial Set, House Reports*, vol. 6 (Washington, DC: Library of Congress, 1957).

176 "Man is what he is": Rudolf Steiner and Ida Wegman, *Extending Practical Medicine: Fundamental Principles Based on the Science of the Spirit* (London: Rudolf Steiner Press, 2000), pp. 11–12.

177 So, for example: "Anthroposophic Medicines: Their Origin, Production and Application," pamphlet published by the Medical Section of the School of Spiritual Science, Dornach, Switzerland.

177 "Illness is a part": Sigfrid Knauer, "The Wisdom in Human Illness," article date unknown; obtained from the files of the Rudolf Steiner Library, Ghent, NY.

177 "He would have a shelf": Interview with John Brousseau.

178 "He was a very sharp wit": Ibid.

178 In her memoir: Devi, *Una mujer de tres siglos*, p. 136; Letter from Sigfrid Knauer to the House of Representatives, April 4, 1956.

178 "one of history's": Jeff Burbank, *Las Vegas Babylon: True Tales of Glitter, Glamour, and Greed* (London: Robson Books, 2006), p. 100.

179 As a wedding gift: William Manchester, *The Arms of Krupp: 1587–1968* (New York: Bantam Books, 1981), p. 783.

179 Devi insisted: Roberto Díaz Herrera, *Mataji Indra Devi: La dama del yoga en Occidente* (Panama City, Panama: Editorial Portobelo, Colección Pequeño Formato, Superación Personal, 1994).

179 Avshalomov was blindsided: Avshalomov and Avshalomov, *Avshalomov's Winding Way*, p. 334.

179 "I begged him to leave her": Ibid.

179 "Knauer, together": Robert Craft, *Stravinsky: Chronicle of a Friendship* (Nashville: Vanderbilt University Press, 1994), p. 189.

180 "homeopathic prescriptions": Vera Stravinsky and Robert Craft, *Stravinsky in Pictures and Documents* (New York: Simon and Schuster, 1978), p. 299.

180 "When you got an injection": Interview with Brenda Barnetson.

180 "His other patients": Henry Barnes, *Into the Heart's Land* (Great Barrington, MA: SteinerBooks, 2005), p. 274.

180 It quickly came to replace: Anne Harrington, *The Cure Within: A History of Mind-Body Medicine* (New York: W. W. Norton, 2009), pp. 143–51.

181 Men, toiling in increasingly: Ibid., p. 159.

181 "The other-directed": David Riesman with Nathan Glazer and Reuel Denney, *The Lonely Crowd* (New Haven, CT: Yale University Press, 2001), p. 25.

181 By 1957: Andrea Tone, *The Age of Anxiety: A History of America's Turbulent Affair with Tranquilizers* (New York: Basic Books, 2009), p. xvi.

181 "Attention physicians": Ibid., p. 56.

181 "Before a new student": Devi, *Yoga for Americans* (New York: Signet, 1968), p. 109.

182 "a propensity for weight gain": William J. Broad, *The Science of Yoga* (New York: Simon and Schuster, 2012), pp. 96–97.

182 Even the most vigorous: Ibid., pp. 61–73.

182 "those involving": Ibid., p. 73.

183 Then, in Bombay: Humphrey Burton, *Yehudi Menuhin* (Boston: Northeastern University Press, 2000), pp. 327, 331.

183 "Freedom had come": B. K. S. Iyengar, *Astadala Yogamala*, vol. 1 (New Delhi, India: Allied Publishers Private Ltd., 2007), p. 29.

183 "I felt that": Ibid.

183 "In recent years there has": Burton, *Yehudi Menuhin*, p. 336.

184 "makes his eyes": "Yehudi's Yoga," *Life*, February 9, 1953, p. 94.

184 In 1954: Burton, *Yehudi Menuhin*, p. 346.

184 "A New Twist": "A New Twist for Society," *Life*, August 20, 1956, pp. 53–54.

184 "I saw Americans": Kofia Busia, ed., *Iyengar: The Yoga Master* (Boston: Shambala Publications, 2007), p. 5.

184 "Many were": Devi, *Yoga for Americans*, p. x.

185 "Yoga is of great value": Ibid., p. xii.

185 "This welcome book": Ibid., p. vii.

185 One reader of: Devi, *Yoga for Americans*, p. 192.

185 "The Yoga exercises": Ibid., p. 193.

185 "Red Heads Turn": "Red Heads Turn for Yankee Yogi," UPI, *Miami News*, June 19, 1960.

186 "The prospect of being": Indra Devi, *Renew Your Life through Yoga* (New York: Warner Paperback Library, 1972), p. 71.

187 "They weren't interested": Devi, *Una mujer de tres siglos*, p. 154.

187 "Numerous Western researchers": Anita Gregory, "Crackdown on Parapsychology," *New Scientist*, February 13, 1975.

188 Some of Romen's subjects: Stanley Krippner, *Human Possibilities: A First-Person Account of Mind Exploration—Including Psychic Healing, Kirlian Photography, and Suggestology—in the USSR and Eastern Europe* (Garden City, NY: Anchor Press/Doubleday, 1980), pp. 244–47.

188 No, Devi assured him": Apostolli, *Indra Devi*, p. 253; Devi, *Una mujer de tres siglos*, p. 157.

188 "Tolstoy is a spiritual giant!": Devi, *Una mujer de tres siglos*, p. 157.

188 This seems to have: Ibid.

188 Foreign Minister Gromkyo: "Red Heads Turn for Yankee Yogi."

189 "Yoga Exercise Fad": Theodore Shabad, "Yoga Exercise Fad in Soviet Union Is Vigorously Attacked," *New York Times*, January 26, 1973.

190 "was of the opinion": FBI memo from SAC, Los Angeles, to the FBI director, June 18, 1962, obtained through FOIA request.

190 "Mrs. HOLLENBECK said": Ibid.

191 "No further investigation": FBI memo from SAC, Los Angeles, to the FBI director, August 31, 1962, obtained through FOIA request.

191 It seemed to Devi: Devi, *Una mujer de tres siglos*, pp. 143–44.

191 "Soon, word got out" Rancho La Puerta website, accessed April 15, 2013.

CHAPTER 14

193 In her writings and interviews: Indra Devi, *Sai Baba and Sai Yoga* (Delhi, India: Macmillan Company of India, 1975), p. 8.

194 "[Y]oga break starts": Kay Goldman, *Dressing Modern Maternity: The Frankfurt Sisters of Dallas and the Page Boy Label* , e-book (Lubbock: Texas Tech University Press, 2013), n.p.

194 "The elevators are motionless": Eugenia Sheppard, "To Be in Fashion, Hang by Your Heels," *New York Herald Tribune*, syndicated in the *Corpus Christi Caller-Times*, Sunday, November 3, 1963.

194 "Problem of Our Age": Devi, *Renew Your Life through Yoga*, pp. 11–17.

194 When she realized: Narayana Kasturi, *Sathyam-Shivam-Sundaram, Part II* (Prashanti Nilayam, India: Sri Sathya Sai Baba Publication and Education Foundation, 1984), p. 257; Goldman, *Dressing Modern Maternity*, n.p.

195 "attempt to stir": "Madame Indra Devi: Crusade for Light in Darkness Has Cloak and Dagger Start," *New Cosmic Star*, March 1967.

195 "On May 12": Letter from the Gloria Swanson Papers, Harry Ransom Humanities Research Center, University of Texas at Austin.

195 Dallas artist Dmitri Vail: Glenna Whitley, "The Art of the Con," D Magazine, April 1992.

196 On the recording: Indra Devi, *Indra Devi Presents Concentration & Meditation*, MACE Records, 1965.

196 "carrying the fire": Devi, *Una mujer de tres siglos*, p. 158.

197 "taken all over": Unknown newspaper clipping found in the Gloria Swanson Papers, Harry Ransom Humanities Research Center, University of Texas at Austin.

198 "Was there, we wondered": Howard Murphet, *Sai Baba: Man of Miracles* (York Beach, ME: Red Wheel/Weiser, 1971), p. 24.

198 "He seemed to lift": Ibid., p. 32.

198 "He is the brightest star": Devi, *Sai Baba and Sai Yoga*, p. 5.

199 She told Natalia Apostolli: Apostolli, *Indra Devi*, p. 268.

199 "Saigon swings": Hugh A. Mulligan, "Vietnam: A Confused, Many-Sided War," Associated Press, March 20, 1966.

200 "He seldom answered": Murphet, *Sai Baba*, p. 54.

201 "This is too much!": Ibid., p. 56.

201 He lived in a dilapidated: Smriti Srinivas, *In the Presence of Sai Baba: Body, City, and Memory in a Global Religious Movement* (Leiden, Netherlands: Koninklijke Brill, 2008), p. 35.

201 "My devotees are calling": Murphet, *Sai Baba*, p. 60.

202 Sathya Sai Baba: Srinivas, *In the Presence of Sai Baba*, p. 55.

202 "We'd sit there and talk": Arnold Schulman, *Baba* (New York: Pocket Books, 1973), p. 94.

202 "wish-fulfilling trees": Murphet, *Sai Baba*, p. 71.

202   "At picnics he": Ibid.

203   Beggars, some with maimed: Schulman, *Baba*, p. 34.

204   There was a small: Apostolli, *Indra Devi*, p. 272; Devi, *Sai Baba and Sai Yoga*, p. 11.

204   Each time it ran out: Devi, *Sai Baba and Sai Yoga*, p. 12.

205   Draped in a saffron-colored robe: Ibid.

205   As she walked toward: Ibid.

205   Sai Baba had an armchair: Ibid., p. 14; Apostolli, *Indra Devi*, pp. 273–74.

206   "both the central communion": Bill Aitken, *Sai Baba: A Life* (New Delhi, India: Penguin Books India, 2004), p. 26.

207   "Away from Sai's": Ibid., p. 27.

207   she found herself growing despondent: Devi, *Sai Baba and Sai Yoga*, p. 17.

207   "cascade of brilliant light": Ibid.

208   Then, when the man: Ibid., pp. 21–22.

208   "Practice Yoga, or the mastery of the mind": *Devi, Sai Baba and Sai Yoga*, p. 23.

209   There seemed to be pearls: Ibid., pp. 24–25.

210   "Didn't Christ feed": Ibid.

210   "He caressed them": Kasturi, *Sathyam-Shivam-Sundaram, Part II*, pp. 234–35.

211   "The greed and selfishness": Ibid., p. 237.

211   "fairy tale": Devi, *Sai Baba and Sai Yoga*, p. 33.

211   "Be happy": Ibid., p. 36.

CHAPTER 15

215   In the early 1970s: Samuel Sandweiss, *Sai Baba: The Holy Man . . . and the Psychiatrist* (San Diego: Birth Day Publishing, 1975), p. 52.

215   "a psychology of pure consciousness": Jeffrey J. Kripal, *Esalen: America and the Religion of No Religion* (Chicago: University of Chicago Press, 2008), p. 157.

216   approached "yogic or 'spiritual' practices": Sandweiss, *Sai Baba*, p. 23.

216   "I had the strange feeling": Ibid.

216   "I had the impression": Ibid., p. 25.

216   She told Sandweiss that Sai Baba had raised a man: Ibid.

216   "You see people like Swami Satchidananda": Sara Davidson, "The Rush for Instant Salvation," *Harper's Magazine*, July 1971.

217   "I felt that observing Baba": Sandweiss, *Sai Baba*, p. 27.

217   He regularly oversaw her classes: Devi, *Sai Baba and Sai Yoga*, p. 38.

217   "All the miracles": Ibid.

217   In 1967: "Hinduism in New York: A Growing Religion," *New York Times*, November 2, 1967.

218   "Chief Guru": Barney Lefferts, "Chief Guru of the Western World," *New York Times*, December 17, 1967.

218 "citizens of *Ozzie and Harriet*'s America": Philip Goldberg, *American Veda: How Indian Spirituality Changed the West* (New York: Harmony Books, 2010), p. 156.

218 He was popular: Ibid.

218 "shit and desire": Deborah Baker, *A Blue Hand: The Beats in India* (New York: Penguin Press, 2008), p. 154.

219 "It brings a state": Quoted in James R. Sikes, "Swami's Flock Chants in Park to Find Ecstasy," *New York Times*, October 10, 1966.

219 "And a second center": Goldberg, *American Veda*, pp. 178–79.

219 "are our best potential": Quoted in Hayagriva dasa, *The Hare Krishna Explosion* (San Rafael, CA: Palace Press, 1985), p. 141.

219 "a loose network of holy men": Jane Howard, "Samadhi and Plaid Stamps on the Swami Circuit," *Life*, February 9, 1968.

220 He told Devi there were too many gurus in America: Devi, *Sai Baba and Sai Yoga*, p. 59.

221 she could use to cure others: Ibid., p. 50; Apostolli, *Indra Devi*, p. 280.

221 They must always avoid sectarianism: Devi, *Sai Baba and Sai Yoga*, p. 51.

222 "Doesn't matter": Ibid., p. 54.

222 They refused to sit separately: "India Will Be Learning Experience: Yoko Ono," *DNA India*, January 12, 2012.

222 "In India you have to be a guru": David Sheff, *All We Are Saying: The Last Major Interview with John Lennon and Yoko Ono* (New York: St. Martin's Press, 2000), p. 129.

222 "He has a high smooth voice": Sandweiss, *Sai Baba*, p. 40.

222 "a great bringer of the word": Ibid., p. 42.

223 "I now wonder why": Ibid., pp. 44–47.

223 "For two years we met": Dennis Gersten, "Holy Madness in Healing," *Psychology Today*, March/April 1998.

224 As a *Yoga Journal* writer described Sai Yoga: Pagés Ruiz, "Krishnamacharya's Legacy."

224 "It was Truth that turned the world upside down": Tal Brooke, *Lord of the Air: Tales of a Modern Antichrist* (Eugene, OR: Harvest House Publishers, 1990), pp. 212–13.

225 "Call me by any name": Tulsi Srinivas, *Winged Faith: Rethinking Globalization and Religious Pluralism through the Sathya Sai Movement* (New York: Columbia University Press, 2010), pp. 81–84.

225 "Thatt vas turrific": Brooke, *Lord of the Air*, p. 213.

225 "Too long": Ibid.

225 "Indra Devi just now tell me": Ibid., p. 214.

225 "of things I had neither said nor done": Devi, *Sai Baba and Sai Yoga*, p. 80.

226 For the moment: Ibid., p. 81.

226 "my friend and companion": Devi, *Una mujer de tres siglos*, pp. 175–76.

226 As she said her last good-byes: Ibid., p. 176.

226 "fundamental virtues": Ibid., p. 72.

226 "spirited away to his home": Quoted in Barbara Betteridge, "In Memoriam: Sigfrid Knauer," *Anthroposophical Society in America* (newsletter), Spring 1985.

227 "Who wants to do a watermelon fast?": Interview with Bettina Biggart.

228 When Knauer got worse: Devi, *Una mujer de tres siglos*, p. 181.

228 "There gathered around him": Excerpt from a report by Nancy and Gordon Poer, *Anthroposophical Society in America* (newsletter), Spring 1985.

229 Without Rosita: Devi, *Una mujer de tres siglos*, pp. 178–79.

229 "For some reason known only to the angel": Betteridge, "In Memoriam: Sigfrid Knauer."

229 "She was so sweet throughout": Interview with Paul O'Brien.

230 "I could never get her": Ibid.

230 "One day she went out": Letter from the Crusade for Light Foundation signed by Shama Calhoun, no date, in author's possession.

231 "all huddled together": Ibid.

231 "because [the money] went straight to take care": Interview with Bettina Biggart.

231 "only the first phase": Letter for the Crusade for Light Foundation signed by Patt Garland, January 1980.

231 "That's the way she was": Interview with Bettina Biggart.

232 He told his wife he couldn't imagine: Devi, *Una mujer de tres siglos*, p. 183.

232 "It wasn't like she was ever going to be sitting": Interview with Paul O'Brien.

232 "One time Baba said": Interview with Bettina Biggart.

232 In her memoirs, she acknowledges: Devi, *Una mujer de tres siglos*, p. 185.

232 "I do not understand": Roberto Díaz Herrera, *Mataji Indra Devi: La dama del yoga en Occidente* (Panama City, Panama: Editorial Portobelo, Colección Pequeño Formato, Superación Personal, 1994), pp. 9–10.

233 "What comes out": Harvey Cox, *Turning East: Why Americans Look to the Orient for Spirituality—and What That Search Can Mean to the West* (New York: Touchstone, 1977), p. 140.

CHAPTER 16

234 "I was caught in his net": English manuscript of Conny Larsson's memoir "Bakom clownens mask: sanningar, sekter och sex," provided to me privately by the author.

235 "She somehow talked to me": Interview with Conny Larsson.

235 "That was in fact the triggering point": Ibid.

236 "felt as though": Brooke, *Lord of the Air*, p. 336.

236 "A sovereign hand": Ibid., p. 340.

237 "She explained that": English manuscript of Conny Larsson's memoir "Bakom clownens mask: sanningar, sekter och sex," provided to me privately by the author.

237 "Many souls on this": Ram Das Awle, "Sai Baba and Sex—A Clear View,"

from the website Sai Baba—A Clear View, http://www.saibaba-aclearview
.com/, accessed July 22, 2013.

237 "[I]t's important to understand": Ibid.

238 "He could go out and murder someone": BBC News, *The Secret Swami*,
aired June 17, 2004, https://www.youtube.com/watch?v=hOjk2NpKMFM,
accessed September 10, 2014.

239 "He was totally illiterate" . . . "Nooooo problem!": Interview with Paul
O'Brien.

239 Speaking through an interpreter: Biographical notes in Indra Devi's papers,
provided by the Fundación Indra Devi, Buenos Aires, Argentina.

239 "Now she's like his new best friend": Interview with Paul O'Brien.

239 Devi adored the ashram's atmosphere: Ibid.

240 One of the lesser revelations: Brooke, *Lord of the Air*, p. 336.

240 Tigrett—who made: BBC, *The Secret Swami*, aired June 17, 2004.

240 This would be difficult: Biographical notes in Indra Devi's papers, provided
by the Fundación Indra Devi, Buenos Aires, Argentina.

241 "Perhaps it is the country's": D. M. Siytangco, "Ceylonese Swami Here,"
Manila Today, January 5, 1983.

241 Devi was embraced: Biographical notes in Indra Devi's papers, provided by
the Fundación Indra Devi, Buenos Aires, Argentina.

241 "There was a great deal": Shirley MacLaine, *Going Within*, e-book (New
York: Bantam, 2010), n.p.

241 "Orbito was left with a bit of blood on his fingers": Devi, *Una mujer de tres
siglos*, pp. 199–200.

241 "She had to realize": Interview with Bettina Biggart.

242 "That was the biggest mistake": Ibid.

242 "I try not to be subject": Devi, *Una mujer de tres siglos*, pp. 199–200.

243 "dying": Ibid., p. 200.

CHAPTER 17

244 "There were words whose": Timothy Wilson, "Starmakers: Dictators, Song-
writers, and the Negotiation of Censorship in the Argentine Dirty War," *A
Contracorriente* 6, no. 1 (Fall 2008).

245 Knowing he was about: Viviana Gorbato, *Vote Fama: El strip-tease de la
clase política argentina* (Buenos Aires: Editorial Sudamericana, 2000), pp.
248–49.

245 "And that": Interview with Piero de Benedictis.

245 Argentineans have always: Michelle Goldberg, "In Treatment: In Argentina,
Psychoanalysis Is as Common as Malbec," *Tablet*, November 11, 2010.

246 In all her eighty-three years: Devi, *Una mujer de tres siglos*, pp. 188–89.

246 "Of course": Biographical notes found in Indra Devi papers, Fundación
Indra Devi, Buenos Aires, Argentina.

246 "[Y]ou have a responsibility": Virginia Lee, "Indra Devi: The First Lady of
Yoga," *Yoga Journal*, January/February 1984.

247 "She loved it!": Interview with Piero.

247 She'd been inspired: Paul Brunton, *A Search in Secret Egypt* (York Beach, ME: Samuel Weiser, Inc., 1984), pp. 68–77.

248 Shama was deeply moved: Interview with Shama Calhoun.

248 "He was like her pet project": Ibid.

248 The trip was a joy: Javier Avena, "Su hija de 90 años," *Noticias*, November 26, 1989.

249 "Will I be there": Interview with Calhoun.

249 During that time: Devi, *Una mujer de tres siglos*, p. 201.

249 "My life with Indra Devi?": Interview with Calhoun.

249 "It was the only time": Ibid.

249 "I had the possibility": Devi, *Una mujer de tres siglos*, p. 202.

250 "adventure and independence": Ibid., pp. 216–17.

250 "She is restless": "Exclusivo: A los 86 años recien complidos, Inda Devi inició sus clases de yoga en nuestro país," photocopied clip from Indra Devi's files, publication unknown.

250 According to Devi, Francesca: Devi, *Una mujer de tres siglos*, p. 216.

253 At that moment: David Lifar, *Las enseñanzas de Indra Devi* (Buenos Aires: Editorial Sudamericana S.A., 2006), pp. 111–12; Devi, *Una mujer de tres siglos*, pp. 218–23.

CHAPTER 18

254 He took tranquilizers: Kevin Buckley, *Panama* (New York: Touchstone, 1992), p. 70.

254 "something I really": Roberto Díaz Herrera, *Mataji Indra Devi: La dama del yoga en Occidente* (Panama City, Panama: Editorial Portobelo, Colección Pequeño Formato, Superación Personal, 1994), p. 5.

255 "an enlightened piece": Ibid., p. 1.

255 "At that moment": Interview with Roberto Díaz Herrera.

256 "Díaz Herrera had a silvery": Frederick Kempe, *Divorcing the Dictator: America's Bungled Affair with Noriega* (London: I. B. Tauris and Co. Ltd.), p. 150.

257 "I didn't realize you": Interview with Shama Calhoun.

257 Somehow, he figured: Roberto Díaz Herrera, *Panamá: Mucho más que Noriega* (Caracas, Venezuela: Cromotip, 1988), p. 69.

257 "My girlfriend opens": Interview with Calhoun.

258 He called her: Andrés Oppenheimer, "Odd Man Out," *Miami Herald*, August 13, 1989.

258 "Oh my God, who are you?": Interviews with Díaz Herrera and Calhoun.

258 *"What good is it"*: Sandweiss, *Sai Baba*, pp. 15–16.

259 "A little session of meditation": Oppenheimer, "Odd Man Out."

259 "He put me up": Interview with Calhoun.

260 "Noriega is your enemy": Interviews with Díaz Herrera and Calhoun.

260 "like military intelligence": Interview with Díaz Herrera.

260 One day, she rang: Ibid.

261 Many years before: Devi, *Sai Baba and Sai Yoga*, p. 42.

261 "Rama, Rama, Rama": Oppenheimer, "Odd Man Out."

261 "What do I do": Interview with Díaz Herrera.

262 "You're going to be bored": Ibid.

262 "Who does Roberto": Ibid.

263 "When a peasant wants": R. K. Karanjia, *God Lives in India* (Bangalore, India: Sai Towers Publishing, 2008), p. 22.

263 "The moment you give": Oppenheimer, "Odd Man Out."

263 "Trilha showed Noriega": Kempe, *Divorcing the Dictator*, p. 210.

264 "You want to begin a total": Ibid., p. 211.

264 "my plan was to make Panama explode": Interview with Díaz Herrera.

264 Finally, he admitted: Buckley, *Panama*, p. 77.

264 "The Godfather's": Kempe, *Divorcing the Dictator*, p. 212.

265 One of these screeds referred: Dan Williams, "Rumors Cover Flying Saucers, Governmental Gossip: 'Lip Radio' Tops Charts in Panama," *Los Angeles Times*, July 20, 1987.

265 "political baptism": Kempe, *Divorcing the Dictator*, p. 213.

265 "It's like watching": P. J. O'Rourke, *Holidays in Hell*, e-book (New York: Grove Press, 2007), n.p.

265 More than fifteen hundred protesters: Kempe, *Divorcing the Dictator*, p. 225; Buckley, *Panama*, p. 93.

265 "In the good old days": Oppenheimer, "Odd Man Out."

266 Priests came to serve: José de Córdoba, "Colonel at the Heart of Panama Uprising Credits Guru in India," *Wall Street Journal*, June 12, 1987.

266 "sits cross-legged": Stephen Kinzer, "Panama Journal: In the Country of the Occult, Power to the Spirits," *New York Times*, June 19, 1987.

266 "I have no doubt": De Córdoba, "Colonel at the Heart of Panama Uprising Credits Guru in India."

266 "He was like a frightened rabbit": Interview with Shama.

267 The colonel: Buckley, *Panama*, p. 98.

268 "For me, Indra clarified": Interview with Díaz Herrera.

CHAPTER 19

270 "above everything": Interview with Piero.

270 "Like some sort of millennial nightclub": Penelope Green, "Modern Yoga: Om to the Beat," *New York Times*, March 15, 1998.

271 Four years before: Kerry Hannon, "Yoga Goes Mainstream," *U.S. News & World Report*, May 8, 1994.

271 That number has since quintupled: "*Yoga Journal* Releases 2012 Yoga in America Market Study," December 6, 2012. http://www.yogajournal.com/article/press-releases/yoga-journal-releases-2012-yoga-in-america-market-study/.

271 When she taught sun salutations: Devi, *Renew Your Life through Yoga*, p. 164.

272 "I was disappointed to find": K. Pattabhi Jois, "Ashtanga vs. Power Yoga," *Yoga Journal*, November/December 1995.

272 Today in the West: "*Yoga Journal* Releases 2012 Yoga in America Market Study."

273 Devi's instructions for pregnant women: Devi, *Renew Your Life through Yoga*, pp. 226–27.

273 "Even a tradition like hatha yoga": Quoted in Anne Cushman, "The New Yoga," *Yoga Journal*, January/February 2000.

274 "I love yoga": Ibid.

274 "Now that women": Bonnie Tucker, "Around the World in a Lifetime," *Buenos Aires Herald*, May 13, 1993.

275 "perceives a great imbalance": Connie Mississippi, "Yoga for Longevity," *Whole Life Times*, July 1993.

275 Saying that it was a "gross injustice": Indra Devi, "An Alternative to Abortion," from Indra Devi's papers, provided by the Fundación Indra Devi, Buenos Aires, Argentina.

276 "Yoga, which was officially taboo": Sophia Kishkovsky, "Russians Embrace Yoga, If They Have the Money," *New York Times*, September 14, 2010.

276 "Suddenly, I hear somebody say": Interview with Tao Porchon-Lynch.

277 "absolute cold-blooded murder": BBC, *The Secret Swami*.

277 "She said there was a crime": Interview with Díaz Herrera.

278 "She was totally in the wrong": Interview with Bettina Biggart.

278 "I don't know!": Devi, *Una mujer de tres siglos*, p. 17.

278 "If you want to rest": Interview with Díaz Herrera.

279 "She was out of it then": Interview with Bettina Biggart.

279 "went in peace": "First Lady of Yoga Dies at 102," Reuters; Fabio Madeo, "Como conocí a Mataji," Instituto de Yoga, http://www.argen-digital.com .ar/sites/yogamataji/comoconociamataji.htm, accessed August 15, 2013.

INDEX